REDEEMING food

finding hope, health, and freedom

laura woodard
R.D., C.L.T.

DEWDROP
PUBLISHING

Redeeming Food: Finding Hope, Health, and Freedom

Copyright 2022 by Laura Woodard

All Rights Reserved. No part of *Redeeming Food: Finding Hope, Health, and Freedom* may be reproduced, stored in a retrieval system, or transmitted, in any form or in any means—by electronic, mechanical, photocopying, recording or otherwise—in any form without permission. Thank you for buying an authorized edition of this book and for complying with copyright laws.

All Scripture quotations, unless otherwise indicated, are taken from The Holy Bible, New International Version® *NIV*®. Copyright © 1973 1978 1984 2011 by Biblica, Inc. TM Used by permission. All rights reserved worldwide.

Scripture quotations marked NASB are taken from the (NASB®) New American Standard Bible®, Copyright © 1960, 1971, 1977, 1995, 2020 by The Lockman Foundation. Used by permission. All rights reserved.

Scripture quotations marked ESV are taken from The ESV® Bible (The Holy Bible, English Standard Version®), copyright © 2001 by Crossway, a publishing ministry of Good News Publishers. Used by permission. All rights reserved.

Scripture quotations marked TPT are taken from The Passion Translation®. Copyright © 2017, 2018 by Passion & Fire Ministries, Inc. Used by permission. All rights reserved. ThePassionTranslation.com.

Cover and interior design by Jay Smith–Juicebox Designs
Hand-lettering by Kristi Smith

Redeeming Food: Finding Hope, Health, and Freedom
Produced by Dewdrop Publishing
ISBN 979-8-9862487-0-7

Disclaimer: The information in this book is not intended to diagnose or treat medical conditions. Names and identifying details of most individuals have been changed to protect their privacy.

contents

PART ONE: A NEW FOUNDATION

1. introduction 11
2. all food is good 17
3. fellowship 23
4. enjoyment and comfort 29
5. celebration and remembrance 37
6. covenant 45
7. honor and sacrifice 49
8. provision and strength 57
9. a reflection of him 65

PART TWO: GET WISDOM

10. like a river 69
11. promise and a poultice 73
12. restriction 83
13. freedom 89
14. seasons 95
15. opposition 101
16. the fruit 109

PART THREE: BARRIERS TO HEALTH

17. divine health 115
18. sin and disconnection 121
19. afflictions 133
20. emotions 149
21. prophetic insight 159
22. a sound mind 169
23. being human 175
24. from glory to glory 183

PART FOUR: THE RIVER OF LIFE

25. two rivers 191
26. redeeming food 197

APPENDIX - WHO IS THIS JESUS?

acknowledgements

To my sister, Lonni: Thank you for fighting for this book with me. I would have given up long ago if it weren't for you. Thank you for knowing how good it could be and pushing me to make it better, even when I didn't believe it was possible.

To my amazing editor, Brenna: Thank you for your encouragement, dedication, and sacrifice in helping me refine and finish this book. Your editorial skills are unmatched, as well as your heart and your counsel. Thanks for getting me to the finish line.

To Jay and Kristi at Juicebox Designs: You have been so patient, generous, and encouraging over the years. Thank you for all your hard work and bringing this book to life.

To Christine Tracy: Thanks for coaching me into the literary world when I knew absolutely nothing.

To my husband, Nathan: Thank you for believing in me, for supporting me, and for sacrificing continually. I love you more than words.

To the rest of my family and my amazing community of friends: My life is so rich because of each of you. You each helped make this book a reality in your own way.

foreword

Time lost in deep conversation with Laura about health, nutrition, wellness, disease, and therapeutics are some of my most cherished memories with her. We were both on educational journeys when the Lord merged our paths in Denver, Colorado. I was in the thick of medical school and she was building her nutrition practice, exploring new ways to help her patients beyond traditional dietetic avenues.

We instantly connected over our shared passion to serve people in one of their greatest needs: when their bodies have failed them in one way or another. Our deepest connection, however, was how we united health to our Creator.

For the last decade, I've watched Laura become uniquely equipped to share this message—as a well-educated and experienced healthcare professional and as someone who has personally dealt with many of the struggles she brings to light in this book. She has spent years asking the Lord hard questions and wrestling through Scripture, while also staying up to date on research and knowledge in her rapidly growing field of study. I've seen this writing process shape her, teach her, and grow her into someone who profoundly understands the heart of God for people, food, and health.

In my own practice in rural Colorado, I ask many of these same questions as I serve those struggling with overweight, obesity, and the resulting medical conditions. Nearly 75% of my patients suffer from being overweight or obese, which isn't surprising, given that 73.6% of all Americans struggle with this diagnosis [1].

Why is this? I've invested countless hours studying years of research for possible causes and solutions, but, when I sit down with my patients and ask the hard questions, there is so much more to learn. Each person has a different story, a different struggle, a different why, and all of a sudden the algorithms and therapeutics—though evidence-based—fall short. Though they are, of course, helpful and often necessary, the person in front of me is more than just a physical body in need of dietary advice, an exercise prescription, pharmaceutical interventions, or surgery. Their needs go much deeper.

In that vein, this is not a book about weight loss but about restoring broken mindsets regarding food and health. I see the desperate need for this in the majority of my patients—to understand the beauty of food held in tension with wisdom. Beyond that, I see a great need for supernatural help that supersedes our human capacity for change.

Laura faithfully puts into words what so many of us have felt in the brokenness of our food and health culture but haven't known what to do with. This book gracefully walks you through biblical truths that will bring you back to the purity of the gift of food while also equipping you to find the balance of wisdom for your health—physical, spiritual, and emotional.

I'm so grateful for this message and for the last decade of Laura's life that has been poured into cultivating it. Her words remind me just how amazing our Creator is, how faithful our Savior is, and the hope that we have in Him.

Amanda Nichols, Doctor of Osteopathic Medicine
DIPLOMATE OF AMERICAN BOARD OF FAMILY MEDICINE
DIPLOMATE OF AMERICAN BOARD OF OBESITY MEDICINE

[1] https://www.cdc.gov/nchs/fastats/obesity-overweight.htm

PART ONE

a new foundation

chapter 1

introduction: why food?

> "God saw all that He had made,
> and it was very good."
> GENESIS 3:31

In the beginning, when God created man, He gave man food. It was a gift, not a responsibility. There were no stipulations or expectations except that man enjoy the gift—a gift to nourish, delight, and connect.

Since that time, our relationship with food has grown more complicated. We see sin enter into the world through Adam and Eve, and the Law of Moses given with all its rules about clean and unclean foods. Yet, even with the limitations of the Law, we still see food blessing God's people throughout the Old Testament, cultivating good things and connecting His people back to Him.

Then Jesus came. His sacrifice on the cross fulfilled the Law—suddenly all that had been unclean was made clean once more. Food would no longer be defined as clean or unclean, good or bad. Eating was no longer governed by laws and rules.

Yet the very heart of our nutrition culture today is laws and rules. We have looked to them to understand why we're sick, and to give us answers for how to heal. We have looked to them to defy aging, regulate our weight, and optimize our health to the highest degree. But the thing about laws and rules is that, though they may help in some ways, they fall radically short of giving life to our spirits and joy to our souls. They fall short of the reality that food is meant for so much more than health goals and responsibilities—it's meant to connect us to the One who formed us and fashioned us, to experience more of who He is and how He loves us.

Food, my friends, is a beautiful plumb line straight to the heart of God. It's one of the most evident ways that we can experience His beauty and taste His goodness in the land of the living. With all the rules and laws we have built around it, our hearts have struggled to hold on to that connection. I think we all sense the loss, to some degree, and we want it back. But how do we get there? How do we experience all the beautiful things God created food for, while also tending to our physical health?

It's a supernatural tension between two very necessary realities, and it starts with remembering, first and foremost, that food is *good*.

"For if a law had been given that could impart life, then righteousness would certainly have come by the law."
GALATIANS 3:21

The first few years in my nutrition practice, I was solely focused on treating the physical ailments of my patients with therapeutic nutrition. Most of them experienced a great deal of success but, over time, I started to realize that the success often came with a heavy cost. Some thrived in strict dietary boundaries, but for others, it was like heaping on one heavy burden after another. I didn't take any pleasure in the fact that making so many changes was hard for each patient, but there seemed to be no better alternative: if they wanted to get better, they needed to make the sacrifices and put in the effort.

I was no stranger to this. For years I had struggled with my own health issues—chronic fatigue, severe irritable bowel syndrome, celiac disease, and thyroid dysfunction—that could only be managed through a very strict diet. Once I finally found answers through nutrition, it affirmed my belief that nutrition is key to our healing and often the best way forward. With every patient who saw their health transform through strict dietary changes, this belief was reinstilled.

Food restrictions gave people their lives back in many ways, but I also noticed what it stole from them. No longer could a meal be merely received with thanksgiving and enjoyed. Simple freedoms like sharing meals with family or friends was difficult—or impossible—for some. Traveling was stressful. Holidays fell flat. For some patients, eating became a solo event—finding it easier to opt out of stressful social situations around food, they became isolated at mealtimes. The protocols began to consume people's lives and focus, and that was never the goal.

There were some patients who loved their new way of eating because it gave them firm boundaries, and those boundaries, in turn, helped them gain self-control. Others came to dislike or resent their restrictive dietary protocols but pressed on for the physical relief they found or hoped to find. Some became fearful of food and how it could harm them. Some became so traumatized by all the diets and protocols that they had to walk away from them altogether. Others became miserable, sad, or resigned to the fact that enjoying food was no longer the point.

Eventually, I decided that seeing physical health improve and symptoms go away shouldn't be the only standard of success we measure. If people were stressed, frustrated, isolated, and miserable, could this really be considered success? Food was meant to be a gift to be enjoyed as well as a tool for healing and health. If we healed the body but destroyed the spirit, were we actually finding the right answers for the fullness of life that Jesus died for?

Diets, protocols, and all that we know about nutrition are good. But, by themselves, they are much like a law—a set of rules designed to control our behavior for the purpose of a desired outcome. But the law does not impart life to our spirit, like Paul tells us in Galatians. There is nothing supernatural about diets and good nutrition in and of themselves. They do not hold the power to nourish both the needs of our bodies and the life of our spirits.

But Jesus.

Jesus is the One who can breathe life on those things to make them good for our bodies and life-giving to our spirits. He is the One who can give us wisdom to navigate our health journeys while also strengthening our hearts and minds.

Good health is valuable. Eating wisely is valuable. But these things are not the only purpose food holds in our lives. For years now, I have watched as the nutrition culture unknowingly lays every other good thing about food on the altar for the sake of health. In doing so, we have also let go of experiencing many other God-given gifts that come wrapped around food.

It is time for us to reacquaint ourselves with the goodness of God found in food. What did He intend it for? How do we partner with Jesus on our health journeys to find answers that are full of supernatural power—imparting life to both our body and our spirit?

Years ago, I asked God a simple question.

"What did You create food for?"

I hunted through scripture to find out what He had to say about food, nutrition, and how we should eat. What I found wasn't a diet; it was His heart. It wasn't about food as a responsibility but food as His gift. The first part of this book seeks to answer that very question: *what is food intended for?* Before we can discern wisdom for what to eat and how to be healthy, we need to shore up our foundation. That foundation is, quite simply, understanding God's heart. When we know His heart for food and for us, our health and nutrition decisions can then come into alignment with what we know to be true about the character and nature of God.

The second part of the book will focus on wisdom. It's the component that brings it all together—embracing the good things God created food for, while seeking Him for answers on how to pursue health and healing. Wisdom is from Jesus, and Him alone. We will explore what wisdom is, how to find it, and what to do with it once you've got it.

We can know if we are walking in wisdom by the fruit it produces in and around us. The presence—or absence—of the fruit of the Spirit that Paul talks about in Galatians will tell us a lot about our food journey and our decisions. They will help us to discern the Lord's voice and the Holy Spirit's leading more powerfully, and raise our physical and spiritual bars for success.

In the third part of the book, we'll talk about different layers to consider with regard to physical ailments. Many people are suffering with health issues, desperate to find answers through nutrition. This is very much in the heart of God to do, but there are times when food isn't the answer, or perhaps isn't the only one. We must learn to discern and understand why we are sick. There may be physical barriers to our health that diet, supplements, and other therapies can heal, but there may also be spiritual or emotional barriers beyond the reach of nutritive solutions.

We will dive into what some of those layers or barriers might be. Rarely do we arrive and remain at a fixed point of good health because health is dynamic and ever changing. In these ups and downs, we will inevitably discover barriers that try to hold us back. We may find multiple layers to our health struggle, not just one issue. Understanding these will help us to discern which steps we can take to find victory. Through it all, we will find the faithfulness of God as we anchor to Him.

As you read this book, I pray you will be transformed in how you think about and look at food. I pray you will be strengthened and encouraged on your health journey, and that the Lord will give you new understanding, insight, and victory. Above all, my greatest hope and prayer is that you will fall in love with Jesus all the more as we unpack the beauty of His gift of food to us in both simple and profound ways.

Enjoy!

chapter 2

all food is good

Just as it was at the beginning of Creation, food is a gift to God's people, and we are free to enjoy it as such. But we also live in a world riddled with brokenness, where sickness happens and health is imperfect—a world where good things can be perverted and undermined.

So when it comes to food and nutrition, what's good? What's not good? How do we measure it?

This is our challenge—to hold on to the good and hold on to God, to let Him teach us the way through each season and circumstance.

With all the noise in the health and wellness industry—ideas, theories, research, trends, opinions, and diets—what do we pay attention to? Even in the Christian sphere, there are enough opinions and interpretations about healthy eating to make a person's head swim. Surely God has something to say about all of this, something to bring clarity. He is not a God of heavy burdens and confusion: His yoke is easy and His burden is light (Matthew 11:30). Does He, in fact, endorse one way of eating over another? Is there such a thing as Biblical nutrition?

Ultimately, what is truth when it comes to food and diet and health? What does God actually desire for us?

The word *nutrition* is never mentioned in the Bible. However, God does have a lot to say about food. His overarching truth is quite simple, but it can completely shift our perspective if we allow it: all food is good and is to be received with thanksgiving by those who know and love God. *All* food.

Let's rewind a bit to help understand just how profound that truth is. The more we learn about health and nutrition, the more we start to label foods as good, bad, and everything in between. Diets are built around this concept. Our nutrition culture stands on it. If I asked you what foods you consider "bad," what would you say? What foods do you believe to be "good?"

What's interesting is that most people will view the same foods differently depending on what they have been told. Those of us who are doing the telling—myself and other health experts—develop our differing opinions because we research through different lenses. A cardiologist will look at foods in relation to how they help or hurt cardiovascular function. A dietitian specializing in weight loss will look at foods' impact on weight, while a dietitian specializing in functional nutrition will see how food impacts each functional system in the body. A dietitian with a passion for endurance sports and sports nutrition will research foods for how they best fuel the body, while a woman's health specialist will look at all the ways diet can support hormone balance and overall endocrine function.

Then you have the consumers—the ones looking to solve health problems or progress toward a goal. Those specific health needs and goals will determine what information they see and how they interpret it.

A person's lens directly impacts what information they consider important, as well as what they overlook, ignore, or deem incorrect. Who we are—our personalities, all our unique experiences, and all that we know—also feeds into our varying perspectives of food and health. Thus, the foods we consider good or bad will almost always differ, and there is no solid definition to universally qualify a food as good or bad.

A variety of opinions can be a wonderful thing, but they have caused a swirl of confusion in the world of food these days. People are becoming ever more aware of how diet can play a role in health and healing, and the pursuit of nutrition has become more common than ever before. We have more information available to us on this topic than we can keep up with, leaving many people frustrated and completely overwhelmed.

What do we choose to believe in a nutrition culture that seems to contradict itself at every turn? When every food can be labeled bad for one reason and good for another? We judge ourselves for how we eat well or fail to eat well, and we feel judged by others who do it better or differently than we do. Where is the standard for right and wrong?

First, let's start with some very basic truths: God is good. He is for us, He is faithful, and His ways are marked by peace.

Peace is probably the last word I would use to describe our health culture today. It feels more like paranoid chaos, in my opinion, which tells me that we have much to learn about God's heart for food and about His faithfulness to us in our health struggles.

Our God is a good Father—a Father who cares for His children, who provides for His children, who protects His children. His expectations for us are not dietary excellence or perfection, but that we trust Him, look to Him, lean on Him, and follow Him. Our health or healing doesn't depend on our striving to figure it all out and make it happen. It depends on His faithfulness and our willingness to trust and follow.

Jesus is our Healer—not food, supplements, therapies, or medication. He can and will use all of these as tools for that healing, but He is the source. We have to learn how to trust His ways and not lean on our own understanding. His ways are not always our ways. They are so much bigger and far better than we can comprehend, and trusting Him is always worth more than striving.

Remember that His yoke is easy and His burden is light. It's not hard, heavy, or overwhelming. So often we adopt a mentality that more is better. We believe that the more we do, the more foods we avoid, the more steps we take, the better chance we will have for good health and healing. With Jesus, however, less is often more. Simple steps of obedience, or actions that partner with faith, can make a profound impact on our heart and health, with better and longer-lasting fruit than what was possible in our own strength.

> "Come to me, all you who are weary and burdened, and I will give you rest. Take my yoke upon you and learn from me, for I am gentle and humble in heart, and you will find rest for your souls. For my yoke is easy and my burden is light."
>
> MATTHEW 11:28-30

In Paul's letter to Timothy, he prophesies about the future church.

> "The Spirit clearly says that in later times some will abandon the faith and follow deceiving spirits and things taught by demons. Such teachings come through hypocritical liars, whose consciences have been seared as with a hot iron. They forbid people to marry and order them to abstain from certain foods, which God created to be received with thanksgiving by those who believe and who know the truth. For everything God created is good, and nothing is to be rejected if it is received with thanksgiving, because it is consecrated by the word of God and prayer."
>
> 1 TIMOTHY 4:1-5

The first thing to note is that Paul is speaking of "later times," or a time in the future—not his present day. It's a prophecy intended to warn the future church of ways in which the enemy might try to lure God's people into wrong teachings, one of which had to do with food.

These verses sound intense, talking about deceiving spirits and demons, but that's because it's important. Our ability to receive things like food—things that God has given to bless us—are things the enemy would love nothing more than to pull the blessing out of.

Paul begins by calling us to an awareness of what the enemy is trying to do—to convince us, God's people, to abstain from certain foods. The truth, however, is that all foods were meant to be eaten with a heart of thankfulness. Why? Because *everything* God created is good. All food is good, whether it is a superfood, processed food, animal food, high fat, low fat, high carb, low carb, gluten free, gluten full, organic, non-organic, or laden with sugar. It is *all* good and able to bless us. The key, however, is our perspective—the lens through which we view and receive food.

"Nothing is to be rejected if it is received with thanksgiving…for everything God created is good." That is the lens through which we ought to look—with gratitude, choosing to believe that food is not meant to make us or break us but to bless us. When we pray and give thanks for the food in front of us, Paul tells us that it becomes something holy, something consecrated. Holy and consecrated things accomplish good, not harm. They are meant to bless, not curse.

When we understand that all food has the potential for blessing, suddenly the fear and anxiety of what to eat and how to eat goes away. It's not that we don't need to learn wisdom or that information and knowledge are useless, but we have to grasp the foundational understanding that food is a gift from a loving God. It is not our enemy. It is a blessing.

Throughout the Bible, food brought joy to God's people. It provided comfort. It brought people together. It was used to celebrate momentous occasions and to show honor. Meals symbolized covenants made and reminded God's people of the wonders He had done for them in the past. In its most basic attribute, food gave strength and nourishment to those in need, sustaining physical life for each and every person. Scripture consistently paints a picture of food bringing good things to God's people above and beyond health and wellness.

I love food. I believe Jesus loves food, and I believe He wants us to be able to love food again, enjoying all aspects of it, while also being victorious in our health. Balance is vital; Jesus is the perfect balance of all things.

Our next few chapters will explore God's multifaceted purposes for food. They will build a plumb line of truth by which we can measure our opinions, perspectives, and decisions. With our plumb line firmly in place, we'll be able to see and experience food as the glorious blessing it was always intended to be.

chapter 3

fellowship

We were created for fellowship and, the reality is, much of it is found around the table. No one can deny that food brings people together. Every culture across the world includes food as a part of social gatherings. It may take on different forms in different places, but everywhere you go people gather around food.

I remember the first time I came to a crossroads between my dietary needs and my love for connecting with people. I sat at the table of one of our favorite restaurants overwhelmed with grief. Up until that point, I had done well with my strict way of eating. It wasn't always convenient, but I made it work and felt great as a result. I had even gotten the hang of travelling by packing all my own food and finding restaurants that could accommodate my dietary needs. This time, however, it was Mexican food—an entirely new challenge. Try as I might, there was nothing on the restaurant's menu that worked. Even the oil they used for cooking was something to which I was highly sensitive.

Several months before this, I had finally found answers to years of health struggles. Those answers meant I had to follow a very strict way of eating at all times. When I did, I felt like a million bucks. After one week on the new protocol, I had more energy than I had had in years, so much so that I didn't want to go to sleep. I felt like I could conquer the world, especially in contrast to years of fighting through low energy, pain, and gastrointestinal issues. This strict diet was hard, but it was also worth it. At least I thought it was. For a few months, I did great. It took work and a lot of planning, but I was enjoying my food and appreciated knowing what I could eat in order to feel well. This was the honeymoon phase.

Then reality set in. The reality that, with most friend gatherings, I felt as though I was on the outside looking in. Holidays meant difficult choices: either inconvenience family members to eat to my standards, bring my own food, or simply not eat. Dinner party invitations provoked a near crisis of faith: to eat or not to eat?

I had become adept at finding creative solutions, but this night was different. We had missionary friends visiting from overseas and it was their last night in town. Everyone voted on Mexican food, and I wasn't about to stand in their way. Once seated at the restaurant, I quickly realized there was no solution to be found on this menu. I looked at everything they had available, thought through all my options, but came up empty.

I was content to forego food and enjoy everyone's company, but how could others enjoy themselves to the same degree when I was not eating? Would it create an awkward dynamic that hindered my friends from enjoying their food and our time together? I could just eat, doing my best to minimize the amount of problematic ingredients in the meal, but then I would likely be sick for two to three days afterwards with severe gastrointestinal pain, brain fog, fatigue, and headaches.

This sparked a deep inner turmoil. *How can I share a meal with others when I know the ingredients will make me sick for days? Isn't sharing a meal together something God created to be good? How do I take care of my body and still enjoy people at the same time?*

This inability to reconcile two realities hit me like a ton of bricks. At that moment, in my wrestling, I realized just how much fellowship and intimacy was meant to be shared over a meal. Food was as much a part of the fellowship as the people, and it felt as though something sacred was being taken away from me—and from everyone around me as well.

I sat at the table completely at a loss for what to do. It wasn't something I knew how to talk about with the others yet and, as a result, my emotions swelled within me so greatly I could barely contain it. Grief, confusion, and frustration flooded my heart and mind until my insides were about to explode. Holding back tears, I pushed my chair back, excused myself from the table, and hurried to the restroom. Once I was safely locked in a stall, certain no one else was in that restroom, I let my shoulders fall and I wept.

Jesus, help me. What do I do?

Tears ran down my face, and then I heard Him speak. His voice was as clear as day. He spoke one simple word that drove away all the anxiety and brought an unexplainable peace:

"Eat."

It wasn't audible but, in my mind, it felt as bold and powerful as thunder.

God washed away all the grief and confusion with that one word and invited me to trust Him for something new. It wasn't what I expected Him to say, yet I knew this was my Father's voice.

I dried my cheeks, walked back to the table, looked at the menu with fresh eyes, and ordered what I wanted to eat. It wasn't gluten-free, dairy-free, or anything-free, but there was not a care in my mind for that. A divine freedom rose up in me, and I knew that there was grace in that moment to enjoy the meal alongside my friends and family.

When the food arrived, we all prayed—over the food *and* my body—and I *ate*. Oh heavens, did that food taste delicious. Melted cheese, doughy homemade tortillas, spicy salsa. My mouth was in heaven. Beyond that, fellowship with friends had never before felt so sweet. I sensed Jesus smiling over me as I ate my cheesy, greasy, gluten-rich meal, delighted that I was so happy and free and able to trust Him.

After the meal, I was in awe. No reactions. Not one. The next day, still no symptoms. Jesus had indeed blessed my body that night to be able to just eat. It was the first time since I started the diet that my eyes were taken off of food as my source of healing, and instead placed completely on Jesus.

I wasn't healed completely—there was simply grace for that evening with friends—but this moment changed everything for me. Food was no longer the ruling factor over my life or my health; Jesus was. Food was a tool, but I would learn to follow Jesus and what He was saying more than my diet guidelines for what I "should" do.

God cares about our health and our enjoyment of food, but He also cares a great deal about our connection with each other through it. We aren't meant to sit on the sidelines but to be fully present, engaged, and listening to Jesus to discover how to navigate it. He longs to speak to us, to lead us, and to help us in those times when what feels right in our spirits also seems impossible in our flesh.

Malawi is a small country in sub-Saharan Africa and, at present, it is the fourth poorest country in the world. Yet, even in poverty, sharing meals holds a central value in the culture. I lived there for two years in my early twenties, and I watched people every day do life around food. Men and women sat in the market together each morning, sipping on plastic cups of hot milky tea and eating flour buns. Around noon, workers everywhere gathered around a small fire, each person with a plate of nsima (maize flour patty) in hand and a pot of vegetable relish cooking in the middle for everyone to share.

From developing countries to wealthy ones, the shared meal transcends economic status, culture, language, and location. It is, and always will be, a place where community and fellowship connect us to one another in the subtle constant of food.

Throughout scripture we also find glimpses of life happening around meals. Perhaps the most significant of them is found in Matthew 26, where we read the story of the Last Supper.

> **"When evening came, Jesus was reclining at the table with the Twelve."**
> MATTHEW 26:20

The last thing Jesus did with His disciples before He was arrested and eventually crucified was share a meal with them. In doing so, He demonstrated the beauty of coming together, unified in spirit, around food. There is so much significance to this meal that we will draw on more in chapters to come, but for now, let's soak in the fact that Jesus ate and reclined with his disciples. It was an intimate moment, one that would draw them closer together, and one that would be remembered for every generation to come.

Dining together with loved ones was the last thing Jesus did before His ultimate death, but it's also the very thing God promises to do for those who faithfully follow Him in their lives:

> "Here I am! I stand at the door and knock. If anyone hears my voice and opens the door, *I will come in and eat with him, and he with me.*"
> REVELATION 3:20

Isn't that profound? Almighty God describes our reward of intimacy with Him as that of sharing a meal. If dining together with loved ones is the last thing Jesus did before His death and the very thing we are promised as a reward for our earthly faithfulness, can we agree that sharing a meal with one another is a very precious and holy thing?

The table is a place of intimacy, connection, and communion and, in our current nutrition culture, this is something we must fight to protect. With all our dietary preferences, beliefs, and restrictions, it's easy to lose sight of this sacred and holy gift—to give up on finding a way. In Part 3, we will discuss more of what this looks like in tension with health issues, but we must first establish that food as a way of connection is the Father's desire for us.

Jesus cares deeply about your connection with others, and He wants you to be able to share that connection over food just like He did when He walked the earth.

chapter 4

enjoyment and comfort

> "They ate and drank with great joy in the presence of the Lord that day."
> 1 CHRONICLES 29:22

From the day we are born, something inside us innately enjoys and is comforted by food. This is good. When a child cries, it either wants a diaper change or to be fed. An infant learning to walk stumbles and falls, then finds comfort in drinking his bottle. A toddler goes to the doctor for some shots, which he finds scary and painful, and then finds comfort in the sweet treat he gets afterwards. Children get excited to eat and delight in discovering new tastes and flavors. Food makes them happy. This isn't something they are taught, nor is it something they learn from their environment. They are born with it. *We* are born with it, and it grows up with us. We can try to unlearn it, but I guarantee that will be a battle fought with little victory.

Food has always been and always will be an emotional part of our lives, meant to give comfort and to be enjoyed. The very fact that God gave us taste buds proves that He wants us to experience our food beyond just consuming it for health purposes.

> "He makes grass grow for the cattle, and plants for man to cultivate—bringing forth food from the earth: wine that gladdens the heart of man, oil to make his face shine, and bread that sustains his heart."
>
> PSALM 104:14-15

Chloe sat across the desk from me, face downcast. "I also ate some chocolate chip cookies," she said. I could hear the disappointment and frustration in her voice as she continued to tell me all the ways she had failed to stick to the diet plan that had been working so well for her.

Initially, Chloe had experienced great improvement with her diet changes. Everything seemed to be falling into place and many of her symptoms subsided. The diet, however, couldn't heal the layers of deep emotional pain that had been stuffed down and locked up from years before. Chloe shared how wave after wave of trauma from her past had started to surface over the recent month. With them came the pain and emotions she had worked so hard to ignore. The rapid physical improvement we had seen in her health all but stopped and some of her symptoms started to return.

The heart will often find its voice and expression through the body and, as it does, it can significantly impact the physical body and how it functions. Facing the emotions of Chloe's past trauma was clearly putting a lot of physical stress on her. Emotional exhaustion made it difficult to follow a strict way of eating because she just wanted to be comforted through food and had no emotional strength left for meal planning or strategic eating. By all accounts, with her health issues, those cookies were the worst things she could have eaten. Some practitioners would even say that this, combined with her other emotional eating choices that month, would set Chloe back significantly in her healing process.

As she confessed her eating "mishaps," including but not limited to the cookies, it would have been easy for me to emphasize the importance of adhering to the dietary changes we'd made. They had already proven to be helpful in the previous few months, so why not just instruct her to get back to it? Why not just focus on holding her accountable and encouraging her?

I could have told her not to eat the cookies anymore. I could have given her other, healthier options or even strategies for how to avoid this emotional eating pitfall in the future. Yet the season she was in was especially hard, and I knew it. It was a season of God healing her heart as much as He was healing her body, and I knew He was not asking her to fix herself by perfectly adhering to a protocol. God is bigger than a few cookies and, in the midst of the pain, He wanted to comfort His daughter. At that moment, strict dietary boundaries were not the answer.

Instead, I asked her if she enjoyed the cookies.

The question caught her completely off guard, but she sheepishly said yes, as though it was a bad thing. I dug a little further. "Were you able to control how many you ate?"

"Yes, I only had two."

"Did you find that these cookies brought comfort to you on a hard day?" I asked.

She thought about this for a moment, and then surprised herself by her answer. "Yes, it actually was very comforting."

"Well," I said, "maybe this is a good thing. God loves to meet our hearts through a cookie sometimes."

I saw the confusion in her eyes but also her slight smile at the possibility that eating a cookie and letting it comfort her could be a good thing. I went on to explain that God created food in a mysterious way—it always seems to connect to our hearts. It isn't wrong to emotionally eat when we are leaning on God. Sometimes, it's His way of loving us. Sometimes, He just wants to meet us through a cookie.

God is the God of all comfort. Jesus is a Savior who is full of compassion for us in every moment and season, and all parts of creation can be a vessel for His comfort. Food, at times, is very much a part of that.

> "Praise be to the God and Father of our Lord Jesus Christ, the Father of compassion and the ***God of all comfort***, who comforts us in all our troubles, so that we can comfort those in any trouble with the comfort we ourselves have received from God. For just as the sufferings of Christ flow over into our lives, so also through Christ our comfort overflows."
>
> 2 CORINTHIANS 1:3-5 (emphasis mine)

Food is meant to satisfy us; it is meant to be enjoyed; it is meant to tend to deeper places of our hearts than we have access to without it. Food is tied to all kinds of emotions. To separate the two has never been God's desire.

In the book of Nehemiah, we read about the Israelites' return to Israel, settling into their own land after decades in exile. Though they had finally returned, the walls of Jerusalem lay in ruins—a tragic reminder of their past sins, which had led to their great demise and horrific exile to Babylon. To return to their city without the protection or honor of walls was unbearably shameful. Nehemiah, with the favor of God and the help of the people, set to rebuilding it.

It took only 52 days—52 miraculous days—and Jerusalem's walls stood strong once again. Its people were home and their dignity finally restored. It was a momentous occasion.

All the people assembled in the square, and the Law of Moses was read aloud. As the people heard the words and the Levites explained the Law to them, they wept. The emotion of the last 70 years came to the surface, coupled with grief of realizing their past sins were what had separated them from God. Perhaps they grieved for all the years of pain and persecution and loss they endured in Babylon. There is no telling just how much emotion was coursing through their beating hearts and thoughts, but we know it was a lot. Now they were finally home, back in a right relationship with their holy God, fully restored.

What did Nehemiah tell them to do in response? He told them to eat.

enjoyment and comfort

> "'This day is sacred to the Lord your God. Do not mourn or weep.' For all the people had been weeping as they listened to the words of the Law. Nehemiah said, 'Go and *enjoy choice food and sweet drinks*, and send some to those who have nothing prepared. This day is sacred to our Lord. Do not grieve, for the joy of the Lord is your strength.'
>
> Then all the people went away to *eat and drink*, to send portions of food and to *celebrate with great joy*, because they now understood the words that had been made known to them."
>
> NEHEMIAH 8:9-10,12 (emphasis mine)

The people wept. For so many reasons, they wept. Their instructions, however, were to turn their grief into joy by eating delicious, luxurious foods. First of all, I love that God's desire was that they grieve no more, that His joy would become their strength. The first step out of grief and towards joy, in this instance, was through food. It wasn't just any food; it was *choice* foods and *sweet* drinks. This meal wasn't about health; it wasn't about moderation; it was about comfort and joy and celebration.

It wasn't the sustenance of the food or its nutritional quality that tended to the hearts of these men and women. It was the taste in their mouths and the fullness in their bellies. We know this seems natural and good but, with our health and nutrition culture today, our minds can struggle to grasp its reality. The truth is, food is meant to be comforting because it connects us to our Great Comforter. Food is meant to be enjoyed and to bring joy because it comes from the One whose joy is our strength.

Patients will often come to me confessing that they are emotional eaters. In my mind, that's a good thing. Yes, emotional eating can become perverted into something unhealthy if we aren't careful, but that doesn't mean emotional eating is unhealthy in and of itself.

Our goal should never be to separate our emotions from food. In my experience, a common reason people fail at diets and dietary changes is a lack of enjoyment of the foods prescribed or an inability to find comfort in those foods when life gets hard or heavy. We were created with an innate desire to experience the delight of a good meal and the comfort of a familiar food. If we don't understand that our natural, emotional connection to food can actually be a good thing, then it can become shameful and consuming—something we feel powerless to conquer. I believe God wants to connect our emotional response to food with our pursuit of better health. It is something He values and something that He wants us to fight for.

Any area of life taken to an extreme, where we deny one part of ourselves in order to achieve a specific goal in another, will not work. It's not sustainable. We are spiritual, physical, emotional, and intellectual creations. We are meant to be all of those things, all of who we are, in every area of life. To ignore even one of those pieces of ourselves for any purpose is an injustice to ourselves and an insult to the One who created us so beautifully.

While it is vitally important to give value to the emotional connection to food, it's also necessary to hold it in balance with discernment and self-control. "For God did not give us a spirit of timidity, but a spirit of power, of love, and of *self-disciplin*e." 2 Timothy 1:7

Self-discipline is often lost when food becomes our ultimate *source* of comfort or *source* of joy. Food, by itself, holds no power to give lasting comfort or true joy. It can only tend to our emotions while we eat it. Once it's gone, our heart returns to much the same state as it was before. This creates a cycle of looking to food to fill a need for us that it really can't fill. In this cycle, overeating and chronic indulgence is common as we can become consumed by our desire for food.

Jesus is the Giver, food is the gift, and we are the recipients. Food isn't the source of comfort or joy, He is. Food is merely the vessel. When Jesus comforts us through food, or gives us joy through a meal, it lasts. The comfort continues to be felt even when the cookie is gone. Joy is felt even after the meal has ended. Jesus gives us gifts that last beyond the last bite.

Chloe's indulgences might not have been within her dietary protocol, but she did not gorge herself uncontrollably. Food was not her source of comfort, nor was it her all-consuming focus and, as a result, she still had self-control. She leaned on Jesus while also working with a counselor and her pastor to help process through her past traumas.

What's your comfort food? The food that makes you feel like you have just been hugged by God? Is there a meal you remember where you felt immense joy through the taste and experience? Have you ever needed the sweet taste of your favorite dessert to do justice to a momentous celebration? All of it connects us back to the One who knows our every thought and heartbeat. He feels what we feel: food is just one extension of His presence with us and love for us. Protect that gift, and steward it well.

chapter 5

celebration & remembrance

Few things in life are celebrated apart from food. It is a part of every wedding, every birthday, every milestone, and even every funeral. Can you think of a time when you celebrated something special and food was *not* involved? Thanksgiving was quickly approaching, along with the holiday season. It's always a difficult season to navigate for people with food restrictions—mentally, emotionally, and physically.

"How do you want me to handle Thanksgiving?" Holly asked. She was, quite possibly, the most compliant patient I had ever worked with, willing to do anything I suggested for the sake of her health and fitness. This question, however, held a tinge of sadness. Sure, she was willing to do whatever it took, but she felt a sense of loss as she considered the upcoming holiday season.

Through blood work, we had identified which foods were triggering her immune system and causing a great deal of inflammation in her body—foods that she was now diligently avoiding. Using additional lab work, we had tailored her supplements to her needs and she was thriving. All the changes culminated in a complete remission of all symptoms, many of which she had been dealing with for years. It was the first time in her life that her blood sugar was stable and she didn't have to snack every few hours to avoid crashing. As an elite athlete, her physical fitness had also reached a new peak where she had become noticeably stronger with tremendously more endurance. She was able to train harder and accomplish far more physically than she had ever done before.

Our goal was for Holly to avoid these foods long enough for her immune system to calm down and her body could heal. Until then, many of the foods she was avoiding still had the potential to trigger an inflammatory response that could make her quite sick, requiring several days for her body to fully recover.

"If I eat whatever my family makes, am I going to set myself back in the whole process?"

It was the first time in months that she had wanted to find a way to go off of her dietary protocol. She just wanted to celebrate the holidays with her family, but I could tell she was extremely nervous about the repercussions. Up to this point, her focus had been solely on feeling good, not sick and sluggish. Now she was considering the value of food in other ways, ways beyond just her health, that impacted her ability to celebrate with her loved ones.

I encouraged her to decide what was most valuable to her in those moments with loved ones: celebrating Thanksgiving with family or sticking to the right foods.

"Thanksgiving is meant to be celebrated," I explained, "and you are allowed to determine what that looks like for you. It's okay to value sharing this meal with loved ones more than your diet."

"Think about the day after you eat," I continued. "God may supernaturally bless you with the grace to eat and not be affected by the foods. But what if you don't feel well? Was it worth it to be able to share that meal and that day with your family? If so, great. Get back to eating well the next day, but be okay with that part of the process."

She completely understood, and I could see how much joy and relief the permission brought her. We're all eager to find this balance of healing and health in tension with the freedom to fully embrace the moments in life where we rejoice and celebrate around food. Friends, let me tell you, it is not only possible, but it is very much God's desire for us.

Celebratory meals and feasts have been ingrained in us since the beginning of time. It is not gluttonous, irresponsible, or unwise. Yet if the heart of celebration is lost, if the love for the people around us is forgotten and we irreverently gorge ourselves on food for the sake of our taste buds and bellies alone, we miss the point. In those times, we forfeit the true blessing of what a feast is intended to be.

Feasts allow us to celebrate and to commemorate significant moments. They help us to remember the significant things God has done. In today's culture, a feast is often understood to be a meal of extravagance or abundance, but if we go back to the Old Testament, where it all began, it was not always about such things. The primary focus wasn't the amount of food or the extravagance of the menu; it was celebration and remembrance. The word feast, in scripture, is often interchangeable with festival because the purpose and focus were not the food, but celebration.

Allow me to take you back in time to the first feast ever recorded in scripture. First, a little back story. God had promised Abraham that he would become the father of many nations and that, through his lineage, mankind would be redeemed. Yet his wife, Sarah, was barren and unable to conceive a child. This was no surprise to God, but before Abraham could remind Him of this huge issue, God gave him another promise to remedy it:

> "I will bless her and will surely give you a son by her. I will bless her so that she will be the mother of nations; kings of peoples will come from her."
> GENESIS 17:16

It was an impossible promise that only God could fulfill. As someone who has struggled with infertility for years, I know just a portion of how weighty this promise is. It probably meant everything to them back in a time when bearing children and ensuring your lineage was your life's purpose.

God was faithful to His word. Sarah conceived and gave birth to a baby boy named Isaac (see Genesis 21). On the day baby Isaac was weaned, Abraham held a great feast—the first feast ever recorded in scripture.

> **"The child grew and was weaned, and on the day Isaac was weaned Abraham held a great feast."**
> GENESIS 21:8

The day was significant beyond measure. The first part of God's promise to Abraham and Sarah, the most personal part, was finally living and breathing in front of them. What better way to acknowledge God's kindness and faithfulness, to express their overwhelming joy, than with a great feast?

Food takes our moments of immense joy and gives expression to the magnitude of what we are celebrating, remembering what God has done. It's difficult to really celebrate something without food. That's not because it's just a part of our culture. If that were true, then how can we explain its presence in *every* culture throughout the world? Celebrating with food is a part of how God designed us, and part of what He created food for.

What is one of your favorite feasts or celebrations that you can remember? Why was it so memorable?

Fast forward to the New Testament, and we find the story of the prodigal son. Jesus tells the story of a father with two sons. The younger son became greedy and demanded the father give him his inheritance. Once he had it, he went away to a distant land and "squandered his wealth in wild living." Eventually, every ounce of money he had was gone, and the land he had moved to suffered a severe famine. Food was scarce—and even more difficult to obtain with no money. He was completely destitute.

Soon enough, the son realized it would be better for him to humble himself and go home to work for his father as a hired man than to stay where he was and steal food from pigs to live on. So he returned home. As the son drew near to his father's house,

> "...his father saw him and was filled with compassion for him; he ran to his son, threw his arms around him and kissed him.
>
> The son said to him, 'Father, I have sinned against heaven and against you. I am no longer worthy to be called your son.'
>
> But the father said to his servants, 'Quick! Bring the best robe and put it on him. Put a ring on his finger and sandals on his feet. Bring the fattened calf and kill it. *Let's have a feast and celebrate*. For this son of mine was dead and is alive again; he was lost and is found.' So they began to celebrate."
>
> LUKE 15:20-24 (emphasis mine)

Notice the first thing the father did when his son returned: he held a feast. The lavish feast expressed just how overjoyed the father was. What if the son had returned, the father had ordered a huge celebration, everyone had gathered, and there was no food? Everyone might mingle, talk, and tell stories but, with nothing to eat or drink, the degree of celebration would have been muted. Anything less than a feast wouldn't have been enough to convey the father's great joy that day.

So many moments are celebrated with food today and, in the familiarity of it all, we can easily forget to look up and soak in whatever blessing that the food or meal is cultivating for us in that moment.

When Holly hit a crossroads where she couldn't celebrate Thanksgiving and adhere to her dietary restrictions, it was as though she was reawakened to the deep value of celebrating with food *and* people all over again. It's just like the old adage of not knowing how valuable something is until you lose it. I think most people today with special dietary needs have become much more aware of the meals and celebrations they took for granted when they could eat without a second thought.

Don't let the familiarity of food, parties, and feasts numb you to the value of what you are celebrating, what God has done, and who you are celebrating with. Remember *why* you feast. If it is a birthday, celebrate what God has done in the past year of that person's life. If it is a wedding, remember how God has brought these two people together, and the life they will live as one. If it is a funeral, remember the value of the life that was lived. If it is a graduation, a holiday, a visit from a friend, or just a day of the week, remember and be thankful. Look up. Be aware of who you are with, soak in the moment, and consider all that God has done.

> **"Be joyful always; pray continually; give thanks in all circumstances, for this is God's will for you in Christ Jesus."**
> 1 THESSALONIANS 5:16-18

Throughout the Old Testament, we often see God tell the Israelites to remember. He knew that we humans are prone to forget, specifically that we are prone to forget all the good things and wonders that He has done. When we forget the works of God, we quickly forget God Himself, our very source of life.

While celebration gives way to remembering, sometimes it's simply the tastes and smells of different foods that awaken our memories and remind us of cherished moments and times gone by. Think about a food that reminds you of home, or a certain smell that takes you back to a specific time or place in your life. We might not even expect it, but one bite, one smell, is all it takes to transport us back.

It's not as grand as a celebration. The value of remembering those moments and seasons may not seem as important as those great feasts, but tastes and smells can be subtle and constant reminders of the goodness of God in our lives.

celebration & remembrance

> **"I am still confident of this: I will see the goodness of the Lord in the land of the living."**
> PSALM 27:13

Memories are important. Remembering our lives—the moments, the seasons, and the people—is priceless. Food enhances those memories in a way that tends to something deep within our souls. Each of us has been marked by food—imprinted at times without even knowing it. It can't be fully explained or understood, but it's just one more supernatural way God designed food to minister to our hearts, our minds, and our spirits.

chapter 6

covenant

"Covenant" is a big word that can mean something both profound and quite simple. A covenant is an agreement between two parties. What makes it profound is who is involved and what impact the agreement will have.

Our lives are laced with profound moments that are sealed with food. Whether it is a covenant between us and the Lord, a covenant between two nations, two businesses, or multiple people, food gives us a tangible expression of the depth and value of those covenants. It allows us to enter into an experience that, if we allow it, will mark us more and more with the Father's love for us.

While covenants can be made between any two parties, the most weighty and profound are those God made with us, His people. The greatest covenant God ever made with us was through Jesus.

On the eve of Jesus' death, He wanted to share the Passover meal with His disciples. This was a meal symbolic of the old covenant God had given, but Jesus was about to become the fulfillment of that old covenant in order to give the world a new one. The disciples didn't know this would be their last meal with Him, but Jesus knew. He knew He was about to be betrayed by Judas, that He was about to suffer in agony and die for the sake of the world. But still, He ate.

> **"While they were eating, Jesus took bread, gave thanks and broke it, and gave it to his disciples, saying, 'Take and eat; this is my body.**
>
> **Then he took the cup, gave thanks and offered it to them, saying, 'Drink from it, all of you. This is my blood of the covenant, which is poured out for many for the forgiveness of sins.'"**
>
> MATTHEW 26:26-28

The night before Jesus died, He issued a new covenant—one that would be paid for with His body and sealed with His blood.

The Passover meal that Jesus shared with His disciples thus transformed into what we now refer to as Communion, or the Lord's Supper. As we take Communion, we not only remember what He purchased for us—forgiveness of our sins, redemption, and eternal life—but, through it, we become one with Him. There is so much promise and purpose in this sacred covenant that we could spend all our lives trying to further understand it, and still never grasp the fullness of its depth and mystery.

It's fascinating that Jesus used the act of eating and drinking to seal up the greatest covenant ever made. This fact alone insinuates that food was created with a divine purpose—with profound layers of depth and meaning.

Communion is not merely an experience of something God has done in the past, it allows us to experience Jesus Himself redeeming us and becoming one with us today. Under the old covenant, God lived *among* His people. Under the new covenant, Jesus lives *in* His people. Each time we take the bread and the wine or juice, we renew our union with Him.

Back when I discovered I had celiac disease—an autoimmune disease where exposure to gluten triggers the immune system to attack the body's own tissues—I started on a strict gluten-free diet. Gluten is a structural protein found in several different grains—wheat, rye, barley, spelt, and kamut—and it is present in any food containing these ingredients. Any and all bread, among many other things, had to go. Any food with possible cross contamination of gluten had to be strictly avoided since the smallest exposure could still trigger a significant reaction. It was a pain to adhere to, but doable. Then came Communion Sunday.

At the time, I was going to a church where they had loaves of bread set out. Each person went and pulled a piece from a loaf and dipped it into a cup of grape juice sitting beside it. All the warnings ran through my mind of what I shouldn't do for health reasons, but I knew the deep value of Communion. It was a sacrament that I simply refused to give up, no matter how broken my body was.

Jesus always healed people. The prophet Isaiah spoke of Him saying:

> **"He took up our infirmities and carried our diseases."**
> MATTHEW 8:17

If Jesus took our sickness to the cross, then sickness wasn't allowed to keep me from the cross. That bread and grape juice was more than just a symbol, it was a representation of Jesus Himself, of redemption, of hope, of life. Surely He would bless that bread and juice to be life for my body, not destruction.

I made up my mind that I would never refuse to take Communion because of my health issues. It was a deep personal conviction. If ever there were gluten-free options in addition to the regular, gluten-full options, I always chose the gluten-full ones. For me, Communion was not a place where I needed to worry about harm or diet. It was for me and Jesus, like renewing my wedding vows with my Savior. Each and every time I took it, my body was able to receive that bread as a blessing, without issue, and my spirit and body were strengthened.

What a perfect testimony of the blood of Jesus giving life. Food is a gift that carries much more blessing and purpose than we realize. If we can harness this truth, our lives will be all the richer for it. Any gift that the Lord gives us is meant to draw us closer to Him, to experience more of His love, and to cultivate rich, fruitful moments for us throughout our lives. It is not meant for harm, only for good.

chapter 7

honor and sacrifice

Food is a universal language of honor that crosses every culture, every language, and every people group. Yet our culture has become so riddled with diets, food beliefs, dietary preferences, and dietary restrictions that it is often difficult for us to just eat what is set in front of us, receiving honor from those who provide it and giving honor in return. Let's look back at one of the first moments of honor through food that we see recorded in scripture.

> "The Lord appeared to Abraham near the great trees of Mamre while he was sitting at the entrance to his tent in the heat of the day. Abraham looked up and saw three men standing nearby. When he saw them, he hurried from the entrance of his tent to meet them and bowed low to the ground. He said, 'If I have found favor in your eyes, my lord, do not pass your servant by. Let a little water be brought, and then you may all wash your feet and rest under this tree. Let me get you something to eat, so you can be refreshed and then go on your way—now that you have come to your servant.'

'Very well,' they answered, 'do as you say.'

So Abraham hurried into the tent to Sarah. 'Quick,' he said, 'get three seahs of fine flour and knead it and bake some bread.' Then he ran to the herd and selected a choice, tender calf and gave it to a servant, who hurried to prepare it. He then brought some curds and milk and the calf that had been prepared, and set these before them. While they ate, he stood near them under a tree."

GENESIS 18:1-8

Can you imagine God coming to you in physical form? What would your response be? The Lord appeared to Abraham in the form of three men, and I think Abraham was flustered. What do you do when the God of all creation appears to you?

Abraham responded by honoring the Lord—these men—the best way he knew how. He invited them in, washed their feet, and prepared a massive feast of food. One seah of flour is about five gallons, or roughly thirty-five pounds. Abraham called for *three* seahs of flour, which would likely have been about fifteen gallons, or around 105 pounds. Can you imagine how much bread that would make? Now, I'm one who always makes way more food than necessary, but this was beyond measure. I guess I would go a little crazy too if God Himself came to my home. Abraham didn't just offer bread, but his best calf, complemented with curds and milk. It was not just a meal of sustenance that he was preparing, it was lavish.

Additionally, to prepare that much bread and to butcher, clean, and cook a calf was no quick task. I love that God didn't come to Abraham in a hurry. He wasn't inconvenienced by how much time it would take him to prepare such a meal. And He certainly didn't *need* that much food. Yet despite all the lack of necessity or convenience, God, in the form of three men, graciously allowed Abraham the honor of serving them in that moment the best way he knew how: through food. The privilege of honor rests on both sides of the meal: Abraham honored the Lord by preparing such a feast, but God honored Abraham in return by receiving it.

I lived in Malawi as a missionary from 2006-2008 when I was fresh out of college. Toward the end of my two years, I was invited to the home of one of our students, Naomi. Her father, Pastor Songwe, led a small, remote village church on the outskirts of town. He was a man we had all come to value and respect for his humility and genuine love for both Jesus and people.

My friend, Barb, and I enjoyed going to Pastor Songwe's church on multiple occasions. The church building—small to our American eyes, but large in the context of what surrounded them—had a thatched roof and dirt floor. The congregation had built the entire thing themselves, brick by brick. The bricks they used were not yet burned to solidify them against erosion, so they planned to eventually deconstruct it, have the bricks burned once they had more funding, and rebuild the entire thing. This essentially meant they would build it twice. Can you imagine?

Pastor Songwe's wife shared with me her dreams of a tin roof for the building—instead of thatch—and talked of real pews to sit on—instead of their split log benches a mere foot off the ground. The church community was poor, but the worship was vibrant and the people were genuinely wonderful.

My two years in Malawi were coming to a close and I had a multitude of books and theological resources that I wanted to give to Pastor Songwe and his wife. I communicated through Naomi to schedule a time to bring my gift to their house, thinking I would just deliver the box of goods and be on my way. As I walked through the small front door and into the main room of the small, tin-roofed home, I was met by their entire family with smiling faces and warm greetings. They seemed so honored to have me in their home, which was mighty backwards because I felt deeply honored to be invited in.

After a few minutes of conversation, I handed them the large box full of books which included Bible concordances, commentaries, and other wonderful materials that I knew were hard for them to come by. It would have been silly for me to travel back to the U.S. with such heavy things, and I couldn't think of a better person to give them to.

As we sat and talked, Naomi was outside cooking. I didn't know it at the time, but she had been preparing a meal all afternoon to feed me during my visit. She walked in with a stack of plates, a pot of freshly cooked rice, and a second pot of egg, tomato, and vegetable stew. I was shocked. It was beyond generous—a lavish meal by their standards—and of course I would not refuse, but it was 3:00 in the afternoon and I was still full from lunch. Plus, I had plans for dinner that night which I didn't want to ruin my appetite for and, if I am being really honest, I was also trying to shed the ten pounds I had recently gained.

I determined to take only a small portion and enjoy it, but then I forgot just how ridiculous small portions are to Malawians. They love their food, much like we Americans do, and small portions are a foreign idea to them altogether. Their lives consist of miles of walking and a great deal of heavy labor. They don't strive to be skinny like many Americans do. Rather, being called fat is often considered a compliment. As such, it was fitting for them to eat such hearty meals. Naomi bent down, scooped out an enormous serving of rice, poured a heaping ladle full of stew on top, stood back up, and handed me the plate with a huge smile. I couldn't help but laugh at the irony of it in my mind.

I gratefully accepted the plate and waited to eat while Naomi served the rest of her family. We prayed and ate, talked, and laughed. The food was delicious and I ate enough to enjoy it, but not enough to be too full. I left a good bit on the plate in an effort not to overstuff myself, but made sure I ate enough so as not to be rude. In that moment, I leaned so heavily on self-control—the very approach we often strive for with food—that I lost sight of just how big a deal this was for my hosts.

When the Songwes saw how little I ate, they were quite surprised. I could tell they had hoped I would eat more than just one plate, let alone three-fourths of one plate, but they graciously moved on. As I see it now, I realize they were a bit sad. This was their gift of honor to me and, while I hadn't refused it, I also hadn't quite received it fully.

I *thought* I had done my best until a few days later when the Lord helped put things into the right perspective. What did it matter if I ate too much, ruined my dinner, and gained a few pounds for a few days? Wasn't it better to just receive the honor and generosity they so cheerfully and sacrificially wanted to give?

All was not lost because I didn't receive as well as I wish I had, but I learned a great lesson through this: receiving honor well actually shows people honor in return, and food can be a vehicle for honor. Honor is a way of love. Tunnel vision can cause us to focus so much on the food, or our personal needs, that we overlook the other values that are right in front of us, such as honoring one another.

In places of poverty, it is easier to recognize when someone is honoring us with food because we notice the financial sacrifice of the gift—it often costs the giver dearly. But as I returned home to the U.S., I realized that I've often overlooked similar moments with friends, family, and colleagues. It never occurred to me that this culture of honor through food is just as important in a first world culture as it is in a third world one. Food is not as much of a luxury for us Americans because, for the most part, we are used to having more than enough. It doesn't seem as big of a deal to refuse food or to be a picky eater because we have the luxury of options and abundance. It's easy to walk into a dinner party consumed by what you can and can't eat, to become limited and focused on your dietary needs.

When Jesus sent out His disciples, he specifically told them how they were to eat:

> **"When you enter a town and are welcomed, eat what is set before you."**
> LUKE 10:8

He didn't give any exception. It was simple: eat. Can you imagine the disciples at the dinner table saying, "Sorry, I'm gluten free/I'm vegan/I'm lactose intolerant/I'm grain free/I'm doing keto. I don't really like olives. I prefer not to eat this." I shudder at the thought, and yet we do it all the time.

When someone invites us into their home and offers us foods we find problematic—whether it's food we don't like, that don't meet our personal health criteria, might make us gain weight, might not be sanitary, or foods that we know might make us feel sick the next day—we have a choice. We can politely decline and, likely, there will not be any repercussions to our physical body. Our hosts may feel a bit bummed that we didn't enjoy what they prepared for us, but life will go on. Or, we can choose to sacrifice our standards and preferences in order to honor the ones who provided the meal. What if we gain a few pounds? What if we feel lousy the next day or two? What if we break what seemed like good discipline after doing so well? What if we get sick? Was the sacrifice worth it?

Isn't the God you serve bigger, and to love people more valuable, than our comfort and safety?

There are two commands that Jesus said were the greatest: love God and love others. Is this not what the suffering love of Jesus is? It serves others and loves others above ourselves, our needs, our preferences. It may be very much in the heart of God for us to honor someone by eating what's given, because receiving the gift of food is just as much a way of love as giving the gift of food is.

When we step out in faith to show honor, asking God for His help, He gives us the grace we need to do so. We might find supernatural grace not to be negatively affected by the food. Other times there may be a cost—not feeling the greatest, or getting sick, or gaining a few pounds—but, even then, there is grace to heal and recover. If we recognize it as a sacrifice of love, it changes everything.

Remember what Paul said:

> "...nothing is to be rejected if it is received with thanksgiving, because it is consecrated by the word of God and prayer."
> 1 TIMOTHY 4:4-5

Sometimes we choose to sacrifice for the sake of love no matter the cost, knowing that this is powerful in the kingdom of God. This act of love affects the person you sacrifice for, even if they don't realize it. God sees. He knows. These moments are very precious to Him.

This life was not meant to be lived eating only the safest, purest, most controlled foods—loving others without risk. It was meant to be lived as a life poured out, loving Jesus and one another through whatever means we can, including the many avenues of giving and receiving honor through food.

Whether our sacrifice is to honor someone by opening our home, sacrificing time and money to prepare a meal for them, or receiving food from someone with a heart to bless and honor us, we must strive to value this exchange—just as God did with Abraham.

I am not encouraging you to put your health at risk in these situations. If you have an actual food allergy—which is different from a sensitivity—or medical condition that could cause certain foods to do great harm, please be wise and very discerning. The point of honor and sacrifice is not to be foolish but rather to gain new perspective and insight to help us steward these moments well. We must discern what the Lord's desire is for us in those moments and then respond in faith, whatever that looks like.

My experience with Pastor Songwe's family was my experience with tons of variables that made it unique. It can't be translated into another person's experience or taken as a formula to follow. The question is: how can you best honor people through the food in front of you in the circumstances in which you find yourself? What is Jesus prompting you to do in those moments? Have you thought to ask?

> "One of the teachers of the law came…Noticing that Jesus had given them a good answer, he asked him, 'Of all the commandments, which is the most important?'
>
> 'The most important one,' answered Jesus, 'is this: "Hear, O Israel, the Lord our God, the Lord is one. Love

the Lord your God will all your heart and with all your soul and with all your mind and with all your strength.' The second is this: 'Love your neighbor as yourself.' There is no commandment greater than these.'"

MARK 12:28-31

Just as food is a gift to us from a Father who loves us, so it should carry a culture of love and honor around it. Don't miss out on those moments; they are powerful in the kingdom of God to bring unity and strength to one another.

chapter 8

provision and strength

God created us to physically need food. Our bodies require it to function, to live, and to be strengthened. With so many diets, trends, and information out there, we often think so much about what we "should" be eating—what foods are good for us and for our health goals—that we can easily forget that *all* food is able to bless and sustain life, regardless of quality or type.

Food starts with the ground, deep in the soil. It requires rain, soil, nutrients, sun, and favor for a good harvest. No matter how much man may, through technology, manipulate the seeds of a crop or alter how it is grown; no matter how the animals are fed and raised; no matter how much the food is then processed after it is grown, God is still the author of all of life and creation. Nothing grows without His provision. Anything that man does, he does with a template of creation to work from.

When you think about it this way, you can see God's creation in every food, from a fresh green salad, to fast food, to a candy bar. Every one of these foods contain creation in them and are thus capable of giving our bodies life. Some foods may not be in their most nourishing form, lacking key nutrients, and may even be loaded with fillers or preservatives, but they still contain some amount of food grown or raised from the ground. Every crop or animal is life that God Himself gave growth to.

If you are starving to death in the desert and someone hands you a candy bar—loaded with sugar, preservatives, and devoid of many vitamins or minerals—would you eat it? Or course you would because, as offensive as it may be to many people, even a candy bar can give our bodies life and strength. That sugar—which was grown as sugarcane—or high fructose corn syrup—which was grown as corn—puts glucose in your muscles and your brain, fueling your body for its most primal functions.

To think about it another way, studies have found that there is a large prevalence of fast food intake for low-income families. Why? It's cheap and can feed a large family on a small budget. Because of this, they do not starve to death. Because of this, in a week of backbreaking work, when bodies are tired and wallets are thin, the family can still eat and enjoy a meal out. Their bellies are full, and they were able to eat something that tasted good. For that, one can give thanks.

A few years ago, my husband purchased two emergency food kits. Nathan is a man who likes to be prepared for anything. When the coronavirus hit and we knew quarantine was coming, stores were running low on food and everyone was in a bit of a panic. I thought about those two totes of emergency food in our closet, knowing that they were far from the healthiest foods and miles from any semblance of my normal diet. In that moment, however, I was grateful for the processed, subpar foods that I would not normally reach for. If worse came to worse, we had food.

These are extreme circumstances, but the point is: all food is provision for life. All food is good and able to be a blessing. All food is worth giving thanks to God for if we understand that food is not our enemy. Every food we despise and cast aside as worthless because of its poor nutritional status might be something we would praise God for if we were in circumstances where we had none.

Many of us have lives where we can choose what we eat, and we know that there is always enough. The beauty of living in a time of such abundance, and with so many options, is that we can eat with new goals—goals that go beyond just enjoying God's provision. We can focus on eating for our health; we can choose what to eat to help manage our weight; we can choose organically grown foods, and we can say no to all the unnecessary things. This, too, is something to give thanks for. It is a luxury. But let us remember that it is a luxury. Let's give thanks in all circumstances, despising nothing.

During quarantine, we never had to touch our emergency food supply. While the stores ran low on many things, we never even came close to going without. Yet there was a fear among many people that stores would run out, that food supplies would run dry, and so people stocked up with cartfuls of everything they could think to buy. I won't lie, I did it too. I bought way more than I ever needed to buy. In fact, there are still a few things in my freezer that were never touched. However, a week into "sheltering in place" God spoke to me very clearly. I was thinking about the next handful of things I needed to stock up on from the store when God gently reminded me that He is my provider. I didn't need to store up for fear of running out because He would always take care of me. He was, after all, the same Jesus who fed crowds of thousands from only a few fish and loaves of bread, with more than they had when they started. He was the God who fed Elijah in the wilderness by sending ravens to bring him food. He was the God who fed the Israelites daily while they were in the wilderness.

He is the God of both seasons of abundance and seasons of lack. In seasons of abundance, we can easily forget that God is providing our every meal, every snack, and even every food we determine we do not need or want to eat. But in times of poverty, of lack, of not knowing what lies ahead and where our next meal might come from, He is the God of those times too. He is the God who provides in every season, though we must remember that His provision is not to be despised for the form in which it comes.

Let us always remember to give thanks. Remember Paul's words, that all food is to be received with thanksgiving. When we say "grace" before we eat, it is a moment to remember our Provider, to think about His provision before us, whether in abundance or lack, luxury or limitation. It is a moment to remember that He will always be our provider, for food as much as for anything else in life.

In 1 Kings 17, God told the prophet Elijah to go and hide in the Kerith Ravine, where the Lord would send ravens to feed him.

> **"So he did what the Lord had told him. He went to the Kerith Ravine, east of the Jordan, and stayed there. The ravens brought him bread and meat in the morning and bread and meat in the evening, and he drank from the brook."**
>
> 1 KINGS 17:5-6

God was not about to send Elijah somewhere and not provide for him to be there. He sent ravens, of all things, to bring him food, and thoughtfully positioned him near a brook where he could drink. Eventually the brook dried up, but that didn't stop the Lord's provision. God then sent Elijah to a widow's home, saying that she would be the one to now provide for him. Food from a widow must have seemed easier to believe God for than ravens feeding him in the wilderness; but when Elijah shows up asking for water and a piece of bread, he couldn't have imagined her response. She had no food, only a handful of flour in a jar and a little oil in a jug. The widow was in complete despair and hopelessness—preparing to use the small bit of flour that remained to make her and her son one last meal before they died.

How confusing, that God would send Elijah to get food from a woman who had none. But if you get to know God, you realize that He does things like this to remind us that He is faithful and, sometimes, to show others His faithfulness as well.

> "Elijah said to her, 'Don't be afraid. Go home and do as you have said. But first make a small cake of bread for me from what you have and bring it to me, and then make something for yourself and your son. For this is what the Lord, the God of Israel, says: "The jar of flour will not be used up and the jug of oil will not run dry until the day the Lord gives rain on the land."' She went away and did as Elijah had told her. So there was food every day for Elijah and for the woman and her family. For the jar of flour was not used up and the jug of oil did not run dry, in keeping with the word of the Lord spoken by Elijah."
> 1 KINGS 17:13-16

Not only did God provide for Elijah but, through Elijah's obedience to go where the Lord called him, He also met this widow in the depths of her despair. Are you where God has called you to be? If so, then there is grace for you to be there. His provision for your season may not be the perfect diet, the most nutritious foods, but how *is* He providing for you right where you are? In the story, Elijah never seemed to touch a vegetable. At first, he had meat and bread when the ravens fed him. Then, with the widow, he only had bread. Guess what? He lived!

We all know that fruits and vegetables are good for us. They contain within them gobs of vitamins, minerals, and antioxidants to support our bodies at a cellular level. Yet God never holds us to a standard of needing fruits or vegetables to live or be strengthened. The life of our physical bodies actually depends on the calories found within any and all food.

A few chapters later, we find Elijah now in complete despair after his life was viciously threatened by Jezebel. This threat seemed to rob him of every ounce of hope and faith. He fled to the desert, plopped himself under a tree, and pleaded for God to take his life. Stick a fork in him, he was done.

The Lord sent an angel to meet him in his despair:

> "All at once an angel touched him and said, 'Get up and eat.' He looked around, and there by his head was a cake of bread baked over hot coals, and a jar of water. He ate and drank and then lay down again.
>
> The angel of the Lord came back a second time and touched him and said, 'Get up and eat, for the journey is too much for you.' So he got up and ate and drank.
>
> ***Strengthened by that food***, he traveled forty days and forty nights until he reached Horeb, the mountain of God."
>
> 1 KINGS 19:5-8 (emphasis mine)

Two profound things happen for Elijah here. The Lord sent the angel to meet him in his despair. Instead of a raven bringing food, or providing through a starving widow, this time God sends a heavenly messenger. The first thing the angel commands him to do in his despair is to get up and eat. This is both provision for his heart and provision for his physical body—the food comforts him, challenging him not to give up, as well as giving nourishment to what must have been a starved stomach. He needed food to strengthen his resolve and his will to live just as much as he needed it to physically survive.

The second time the angel speaks, he tells Elijah now to eat for the journey ahead. It wasn't for sustenance or comfort alone this time, but to store up strength for what was ahead—strength for physical stamina as well as strength of heart to endure. That cake of bread sustained Elijah for an entire 40-day journey. It wasn't just 40 days of survival but 40 days of walking, hiking, and climbing to get to the mountain of God. It was 40 days of not giving up, of hanging on to hope, of choosing to trust the Lord. When God provides food, when His blessing is on it, no matter the food, it can actually accomplish far more than it naturally should.

God can bless any food to nourish you beyond its intrinsic nutritional value. Instead of a superfood, perhaps consider it a supernatural food.

Consider this when you, for whatever reason, do not have the options of eating to a standard you think you should. Do you believe God can bless it to nourish and sustain you just as He did with Elijah? The key is simply to be thankful for it, recognizing it as His gift and provision.

God gives us the grace we need to be where He calls us to be and to go where He calls us to go. If you need His grace, it is there for you. If you need His wisdom to figure out a better way within your circumstances, He can give that to you, too.

Remember:

> **"All that we eat is made sacred by the word of God and prayer."**
> 1 TIMOTHY 4:5 (TPT)

During the Q&A portion of one of my speaking engagements, a soft-spoken woman—likely in her 60s—raised her hand. I could tell she was deep in thought, plagued with curiosity about so many things she had never considered in regard to food. I pointed to her raised hand, eager to hear her question.

"I'm on a fixed income," she started. "I want to buy organic foods and all the foods I know are best for me, but I just can't afford them. Do you have any advice?"

I love these types of questions because I see people finally trying to reconcile everything they know about nutrition with the heart of God and the reality of their circumstances.

"I don't believe that we are doomed by our circumstances," I began. "If you can't afford organic foods, what can you afford? Celebrate what you can do, and ask God to bless it."

She nodded slightly, with a bit of relief, but wanting to understand more.

I continued. "If we serve a God who can move mountains, a God who can provide for Elijah in the desert with ravens, a God who can heal the sick and raise the dead, then don't you think He is also a God who can take something that we give thanks for and bless it to nourish us more than we think it naturally should?"

Wheels were turning in everyone's minds at this point, and I had to make my point clear.

"In 1 Timothy 4, Paul writes that all food is made holy, or sacred, by the word of God and prayer. The key to this is thanksgiving." I paused for a moment, making sure everyone was tracking before continuing on. "God meets us where we are, wanting us to simply acknowledge His provision in those seasons, to give thanks, and allow Him to bless that food to be supernaturally good to us."

The God we know to be almighty and all-powerful in other areas of our lives is just as mighty and powerful when it comes to food and our health. It's easy to put God in a box with health and nutrition, but that's not where He wants to be.

The key here is not what or how you eat, it's the simple understanding that God, Creator of heaven and earth, provides for you. Don't despise the lesser things. Don't hold so fast to the standards the world gives for our diet that we can't be grateful for provision as it comes, in whatever form it takes. There is grace for you to be healthy and blessed, even in imperfect circumstances and seasons.

chapter 9

a reflection of him

Hopefully by now, you see how food—and what we do with it—has the ability to reflect the very character of God in our lives. It is a vessel through which He loves us and blesses us in ways beyond measure. As such, we need to protect the heart of that gift on all levels.

Our pursuit of health should not take such precedence in our lives that they begin to look nothing like Jesus or His ways. Nor should we neglect it, taking it for granted. Rather, our decisions with food—whether in moments, meals, celebrations, or seasons—ought to measure up to a standard of truth that can be upheld by both the word of God and the character of God. How we steward the gift of food in our lives should ultimately carry the same values as heaven. If those values start to fade for any reason, we must recognize that somewhere along the way we have departed from the heart of the gift and the heart of the Father who gives it.

The gift is not meant to be hard or to be so deep and spiritual that we are constantly contending to attain it. But it's a new way of thinking—a new way of seeing—that looks at food from a heavenly perspective as well as an earthly one. It seeks to break off old mindsets and retrain our way of thinking about food and health to one full of hope and life. Our culture has taken a huge interest in food and nutrition and, as a result, we have a lot of opinions, trends, and information telling us what's good and bad, right and wrong, and what we should do. But our standard isn't the world's understanding or formulas. Our standard is one of truth, seeing food as a gift that reflects the heart and nature of the God who provides it.

This foundation of truth starts with simply remembering that all food is good and intended for blessing. Food is a gift that reflects the heart of the Father, and He is redeeming it to become that gift once more.

As we move on to learning about wisdom for our health, we will find that wisdom will stand on and uphold these truths; it will not supplant them. Wisdom is breathed out from the heart and mind of God. It bears the resemblance of His character and will always reflect who He is and what He values.

PART TWO

get wisdom

chapter 10

like a river

> "Get wisdom, get understanding; do not forget my words or swerve from them. Do not forsake wisdom, and she will protect you; love her, and she will watch over you. Wisdom is supreme; therefore get wisdom. Though it cost you all you have, get understanding."
>
> PROVERBS 4:5-7

The simple truth about food and health: there is no perfect formula for every person, and there is no perfect formula for every situation. But there is wisdom.

Wisdom is not simply knowing what to do or what to eat. It's not about right and wrong, good or bad. Wisdom comes directly from the heart of God, and it is given for the good of His people. It—or as Solomon says in Proverbs, "she"—can only come from Jesus.

Rules and diets cannot impart life. That's why so many of us are dying in our health journeys—we've become slaves to the rules and protocols. They are a heavy yoke to carry on our own, and it can feel like they are sucking the life out of us instead of giving life to us. Jesus' ways are bigger than a formula, and we are far more complex and beautiful than a formula has the capacity for.

Wisdom, therefore, is not a fixed set of boundaries or rules. It is like a river that ebbs and flows. It will look different from season to season, from day to day, and from moment to moment. A river never looks the same or flows the exact same way in two different places or at two different times because it bends and turns, ebbs and flows, swells and shrinks based on an infinite number of variables.

Since wisdom is ever changing like a river, we have to be connected to the Source so that we can readily discern how to live in it. Our intimacy with Jesus is the key. We don't just use Him for answers, going to Him for a handout when we are desperate. He will meet us in our desperation but, ultimately, He wants our hearts—our connection. From that place of connection, He speaks, He answers, He helps us, He leads us. It's why rules will never be enough; because if they were, He would be doing us a great injustice.

The first step toward wisdom for food and health is to get back to our first love—Jesus. From this place of relationship with our Savior, we can truly hear His voice and know His leading. If you have wandered from Him for any reason, settle back into His heart. Reconnect with your Savior and let Him minister to you. From that place, answers flow as freely as a river, imparting life to every part of who you are.

How we eat, what we eat, why we eat, and the decisions we make for our health ought to come from wisdom. Anything less will not do. To find wisdom, we must ask for it. If we are physically disciplined and well informed with worldly knowledge yet spiritually passive—naive to what God is saying and doing—true wisdom will elude us. That's because wisdom doesn't come from knowledge and discipline; it comes from Jesus and His Holy Spirit. It provides the way for discernment in each circumstance, moment, or season.

Does this mean that research and learning, diets and self-discipline are worthless? Not at all. But wisdom takes all the knowledge and information in front of us and filters it through the heart of God to discern what is good and right in that moment. What is He breathing on? What is He *not* breathing on? Wisdom doesn't take action first and then consult the Lord for His blessing later. It seeks the Lord first, then moves forward with discernment. It upholds both the need to hear from the Lord, the need for His supernatural help, the need for knowledge and understanding, and the need to act.

Wisdom from God is always creative and unique. Its solutions are beyond the naked eye, never an exact replica of someone else's journey, nor a replication of a previous season in our journey. Wisdom is fresh, personal, and profound. It's not hard or heavy but, as Jesus says, its yoke is easy and its burden is light. Though the journey may require effort for us to follow wisdom's ways, the Lord's grace always accompanies it, enabling us to persevere and endure with peace.

How can we know if we are walking in wisdom? By the truth and by the fruit. Whatever decisions we make with our food, our diets, and our health journeys, ought to line up with the character of God—the truth of who He is and His Word—and then bear fruit in us that is full of life—the fruit of the Spirit. What is the fruit of the Spirit?

> **"But the fruit of the Spirit is love, joy, peace, patience, kindness, goodness, faithfulness, gentleness, and self-control..."**
> GALATIANS 5:22-23

Would you describe your health journey or your outlook on food by any of these adjectives—love, joy, peace, patience, kindness, goodness, faithfulness, gentleness, and self-control? Or, do you find any of the opposite things coming out of you—shame, hatred, selfishness, resentment, anxiety, fear, lack of peace, frustration, negativity, instability, harshness, or compulsion? The fruit tells us a lot about the source from which we are functioning—whether it's from the Spirit or from our flesh.

Remember that, while the physical remission of symptoms and attaining health goals are important indicators, they are not the primary standard of measure we need to be looking at. If we are walking in wisdom, we will begin to see her abundant fruit in every area of our lives—including our physical health. As we learn to walk in wisdom, Jesus will lead us to the answers and victories we are contending for. Wisdom is the way to healing and overcoming. Wisdom is the way to health and thriving.

As we expound more on godly wisdom in this section of the book, the truth and the fruit will be our anchor—painting a heavenly standard for our journey. As Solomon says, wisdom will protect us and watch over us so that we may fully live.

chapter 11

promise and a poultice

> *"...for I am the Lord, **who heals you**."*
> EXODUS 15:26 (emphasis mine)

Jehovah Rapha—the "God who heals." He is the Lord who restores. It's who He is. How that plays out in our lives will look different for each person, but it's so valuable to first understand that the God of all creation is *for* you, and He is with you in your health journey.

God can heal or help us in a miraculous moment. He can lay the answers we need at our feet at any point in time. In fact, He delights in doing these things. But there are also times when He doesn't just want to do things for us, He wants to do things *with* us.

It's easy to jump straight to the "Jesus, heal me" or "Jesus, fix me" prayer without first considering what God has to say about it all. When a healing miracle doesn't come instantly, when answers seem hidden and the odds feel impossible, perhaps it is God's fatherly love drawing us to come to Him for answers, strategies, and solutions that only He can give. This requires both faith to hear and then wisdom to act. Whatever He speaks or however He leads may change our entire understanding of our situation or the entire trajectory in which we move forward. Hearing and discerning is the first step of faith.

We can easily skip going to God for help and trudge forward in our own strength and devices. We can focus so much on doing that we lose sight of what God is saying or we can focus so intensely on what God is saying that we never act. What if we found the beautiful unity that's possible between the Lord's voice and our efforts, where both are of great value?

In 2 Kings, Hezekiah overcame the illness that was supposed to take his life—one of my favorite stories.

> **"In those days Hezekiah became ill and was at the point of death. The prophet Isaiah son of Amoz went to him and said, 'This is what the Lord says: "Put your house in order, because you are going to die; you will not recover."'**
>
> **Hezekiah turned his face to the wall and prayed to the Lord, 'Remember, O Lord, how I have walked before you faithfully and with wholehearted devotion and have done what is good in your eyes.' And Hezekiah wept bitterly.**
>
> **Before Isaiah had left the middle court the word of the Lord came to him: 'Go back and tell Hezekiah, the leader of my people, "This is what the God of your father David says: I have heard your prayer and seen your tears; I will heal you. On the third day from now you will go up to the temple of the Lord. I will add fifteen years to your life. And I will deliver you and this city from the hand of the king of Assyria. I will defend this city for my sake and for the sake of my servant David."' Then Isaiah said, 'Prepare a poultice of figs.' They did so and applied it to the boil, and he recovered."**
>
> 2 KINGS 20:1-7

When Hezekiah first became ill, the Lord sent Isaiah to tell Hezekiah about this illness. I don't know if Hezekiah asked the Lord, or if God just spoke of His own volition, but either way it was mightily important that Hezekiah heard from God to understand what was happening. Then he could respond accordingly.

We all have our choice in how we respond to what God says, but we need to pause and listen to what He has to say first. Then we can respond to what is actually true, not just what first appears to be true.

In response, Hezekiah chose to plead with God for mercy. He chose to remind God of his life of wholehearted devotion to Him, then left the rest in God's hands.

The Lord responded with a promise, "I will heal you...I will add fifteen years to your life." Once the promise was given, Isaiah proceeded to prescribe physical treatment by ordering a poultice of figs to be applied to his boil. The poultice of figs was the medicine used, but it is not the source of healing in this story—God is.

It would be tempting to take that promise and just wait for God to do it. After all, He said it; surely He would do it. So why the poultice of figs? Because sometimes God wants us to do something to partner with the promise to bring it to pass. This action is not a lack of faith but an agreement in faith.

Once the promise was made, Isaiah acted. Isaiah's instructions to apply a poultice seem silly when the God of all creation just promised to heal Hezekiah, but it wasn't. This was their act of faith to agree with that promise. The medicinal poultice was then effective *because* of the promise. God loves to do supernatural things through natural means. Yet without inquiring of God—without the promise—the poultice would have been useless. Hezekiah would have died, no matter the treatment.

If Hezekiah hadn't heard from God first, he wouldn't have known to ask for mercy. Without Hezekiah's response in prayer, God wouldn't have shown great mercy, Isaiah's poultice of figs wouldn't have accomplished much, and Hezekiah's life would have ended. Hearing what God has to say changes everything.

We don't have to be on our deathbed to cry out to God for healing; it doesn't have to be a severe health condition that warrants the help of the Almighty. It could be for weight loss, more energy, clearer skin, self-control, or healing from any sort of health issue. Whatever the case, God cares about the big and small things in our world because He cares about us. He actually wants to speak, to give us greater insight and understanding; but His voice is one that, more often than not, needs to be sought out and tuned into. We can easily miss it if we aren't paying attention.

Lean in to Jesus for all that you need. No matter how big or small, seek Him to know what He is saying. It isn't always as audible and clear as it was with Hezekiah, but He will answer.

Ask for a promise. Ask for revelation. *God, what are you saying?*

Once God speaks, you can stand on it, lean on it, and remember it when you need its strength. You can use it as ammunition when you pray—God loves to be reminded of His promises, and we often need to remind ourselves. If your journey is longer than you expected or hoped, revelation from Him will help keep hope alive.

You might discern in your spirit what God's wisdom is for you; He may speak to you through His Word. It may come through a dream, a vision, an impression on your spirit and mind, another person, a scripture, or any number of ways. We can't always anticipate how He will speak to us or lead us until He does, but we can be certain that He speaks to those who are willing to listen, and His sheep will know His voice. We will know His voice.

> **"My sheep listen to my voice; I know them and they follow me."**
> JOHN 10:27

Once you have that promise or revelation, then you can determine how to respond. How do you feel led to partner with the words He spoke? Do you feel a call to wait on Him and contend, or do you feel prompted to act and take certain steps? What is He highlighting for you to partner with Him?

God loves to give us understanding, to speak promises, and to bless our poultices. It's a beautiful and mysterious tension of learning to operate in both godly discernment and the world's knowledge to find divine wisdom. If we don't recognize that the tension is meant to be there, we can lean so far into faith that we neglect doing anything at all, or we can lean so far into "doing our part" that we overburden ourselves with more than God ever wanted us to carry. It's the old challenge of faith versus works.

In the last decade of working with patients, I often found that I was the second, fourth, or even tenth practitioner that some patients had been to for answers. Many had also consulted with "Dr." Google, numerous health books, blogs, and health-conscious friends for answers before coming to me. You could see the wear on their faces, having tried diet after diet, supplement after supplement, medications, therapies, and the like, and still not having found the health and healing they were looking for.

We live in a world inundated with information, with all sorts of people trying to give us answers. We can easily fall into a vicious cycle of chasing after the wind—doing all the right things and yet still remaining sick. It's not that the information is wrong, that the supplement is bad, that the practitioner doesn't know what they are doing, that the therapies are flawed. But perhaps it wasn't the right thing. Perhaps it was the wrong poultice; or maybe the right poultice but without the promise and blessing needed for it to become powerful and effective to heal.

It's important, in these times, that we seek to hear from the Lord with clarity. Jesus only did what He saw the Father doing and, as such, we need to be intentional to do the same. When the Lord speaks, His voice carries such clarity that even His quiet whisper can silence the noise of a thousand raging voices around us. Noise will torment and confuse, but the voice of the Father comforts and directs.

In 2 Kings we find the story of Naaman, a great commander for the king of Aram's army who suffered from leprosy. His troops had taken a young girl from Israel captive and made her a servant for Naaman's wife. When the young Jewish girl saw his affliction, she urged him to go see the prophet, Elisha, who could cure him.

Eventually Naaman shows up at Elisha's door with his horses and chariots. Elisha sends him a message saying, "Go, wash yourself seven times in the Jordan, and your flesh will be restored and you will be cleansed." 2 Kings 5:10

Naaman was indignant at the instructions.

> "...'I thought he would surely come out to me and stand and call on the name of the Lord his God, wave his hand over the spot and cure me of my leprosy. Are not Abana and Pharpar, the rivers of Damascus, better than any of the waters of Israel? Couldn't I wash in them and be cleansed?' So he turned and went off in a rage."
>
> 2 KINGS 5:11-12

How many times do we think we know what we need? Or we expect God to answer in some great fanfare, but instead He speaks differently, leading us in ways that we don't like.

> "Naaman's servants went to him and said, "My father, if the prophet had told you to do some great thing, would you not have done it? How much more, then, when he tells you, 'Wash and be cleansed'!" So he went down and dipped himself in the Jordan seven times, as the man of God had told him, and his flesh was restored and became clean like that of a young boy."
>
> 2 KINGS 5:13-14

Because God's instructions came in a package he didn't expect, with instructions that didn't seem to make sense, Naaman almost missed out on being healed. I laugh to think how He wanted some great fanfare and to be told to do some great thing to gain the miracle, but the reality of the request was much simpler and more humble.

Also bear in mind that, had Naaman gone to wash seven times in the Jordan on his own—without having heard from God through the prophet—it wouldn't have worked. Why? Because it wasn't about the act itself but about partnering with God, Jehovah Rapha. He made the action powerful and effective to heal.

We must pay attention when God speaks and follow as He leads. He values our obedience, not pointless sacrifice.

> "...'Does the Lord delight in burnt offerings and sacrifices as much as in obeying the voice of the Lord? To obey is better than sacrifice'..."
> 1 SAMUEL 15:22

So many people have given up numerous foods and sacrificed tremendously for the sake of their health, all in their own strength and understanding. This doesn't please God, and there is no supernatural power in it to accomplish something greater. We may think we need to do big things with our diet in order to partner with the Lord or to achieve health, but His ways might very well be simpler than we expect. His leading may ask us to be more humble than we are prepared for. On the flip side, we may think we need to do very little, but He asks us to take a giant step that is way outside our comfort zone or what we expected.

To obey is better than all the sacrifice we can muster. Because Naaman finally obeyed, he was healed and cleansed. Wisdom is prudent. It is cautious and discerning. It doesn't yield to every new wave of teaching or strive for every potential solution. It listens first, then discerns, and then it acts. This is opposite to our human tendency that prompts us to action first, inquiring of the Lord for His blessing or insight second.

On the flip side, I have had patients who are full of faith in God's supernatural power, certain that He will heal them. In response, they will pray, seek prayer from others, hold tight to prophetic words, and listen for all the promises God has. They yearn to hear from God, yet they will only commit to doing so much for themselves because doing too much feels as though they aren't trusting God—they are full of faith, but lacking in works.

Both ends of the pendulum are missing something of great value: faith and action go hand in hand. Without faith, the poultice might not be effective. Without the poultice, faith might never be activated.

> "...faith by itself, if it is not accompanied by action, is dead."
> JAMES 2:17

> "You see that his faith and his actions were working together, and his faith was made complete by what he did."
> JAMES 2:22

Jesus wants to partner with us on our journey because there is something richly powerful in learning to operate together as one with our Savior—learning how to listen, how to respond, and when and how to act. Jesus doesn't want a one-sided relationship, but one where we can abide fully in Him.

Katie reached out to me a year after God had miraculously healed her of celiac disease. Even though the celiac was gone, Katie was still struggling with her health and didn't know how to get better. She was eating whatever she wanted—no restrictions, no boundaries—because God had healed her. As she saw it, she was standing in faith by eating anything she wanted. Eventually, standing in faith wasn't enough, and she reached out to me for help.

I worked with Katie to discover what was going on in her body and what it needed in this new season. She made the necessary changes to her diet, and her health dramatically improved.

A few months later, she went to a prayer service and was certain God had healed her—this time, of *everything*. He had spoken a promise to her and in response, she felt she no longer needed to worry about what she was eating or do anything to practically support her health. Instead she was convinced to stand solely in faith. Sure enough, a year later she was back in my office with the same health issues.

It wasn't that God wasn't speaking, or even that He wasn't healing her. To her, she either had to do everything for her health, relying on what felt like her own devices, or she threw it all out to stand in faith and trust God's promises. She couldn't yet grasp that, while the Lord may have been healing her—whether it was a promise of healing to come, or a declaration of healing that was already happening—there were also things He wanted her to do to partner with that.

Once she understood the idea of partnering with the promises God had spoken for her health, she was ready to get back to eating what her body needed. This time she decided not to do everything she could or should do but instead focus on making the few changes she felt were wise for her in this season. As a result, her health stabilized as did her heart. She no longer swung from one end of the pendulum to the other and no longer felt overwhelmed by it all.

Katie did well at that point and her health stabilized for years to come. As seasons changed and her health ebbed and flowed, she grew in discernment to know what to do and where to go for answers. She knew the nudge of the Lord that would propel her to act, as well as the peaceful embrace of the Lord that told her to wait. She learned to seek the Lord for what He had to say, then to discern what information was right and good for her and what was not—what advice to heed, and what to let go of.

Partnering with the Lord requires that we pay attention and respond accordingly. He may give us specific steps to take, or He may just give us greater insight and understanding. A poultice doesn't have to be a prescription from the Holy Spirit telling us exactly what we need to do, though it might be. The Lord never told Isaiah to apply a poultice of figs specifically. Rather, the poultice of figs was the prescribed treatment of that day and age, and it was given in accordance with what the Lord was doing.

Sometimes there is a right path the Lord is marking out for us, but sometimes there is no right or wrong. It's just hearing and responding in agreement—in faith.

Wisdom doesn't involve striving. If, in your actions, you find yourself striving—desperately trying anything and everything to find how to partner with what God is saying—you have stepped out of abiding in Him. Striving is the fruit of our flesh. Peace is the fruit of the Spirit. Our actions should produce peace. They should feel as though they line up with what He has spoken.

There simply is no rest for our spirit or souls in solutions and actions alone. When they fail to produce the desired result, we will only grasp for something else to hold onto. But we find true rest in the promises and revelation of God, in the nearness and blessing of Jesus, our Healer. This type of rest is one for our spirits, and it comes whether or not our actions produce the desired result.

Jesus does not waver and will be faithful to His Word. If one step doesn't work out, just continue on the journey. Step back every so often, and make sure your decisions and actions are still marked by His peace. Pay attention to anything specific the Lord might be giving you to do. But remember to put your trust in His faithfulness, not the effectiveness of any diet, protocol, or treatment.

When we put Him first and stay in step with Him, His blessing will surely follow in the steps we take.

> "So do not worry, saying, 'What shall we eat?' or 'What shall we drink?' or 'What shall we wear?'" For the pagans run after all these things, and your heavenly Father knows that you need them. But seek first his kingdom and his righteousness, and all these things will be given to you as well."
>
> MATTHEW 6:31-33

> "Become intimate with Him in whatever you do, and He will lead you wherever you go. Don't think for a moment you know it all, for wisdom comes when you adore Him with undivided devotion and avoid everything that is wrong. Then you will find the *healing refreshment your body and spirit long for.*"
>
> PROVERBS 3:6-7 (TPT, emphasis added)

chapter 12

restriction

I met my husband not long after I started on my very restrictive way of eating. The first time I told him the list of foods I couldn't eat, his jaw dropped. He'd never known anyone to have food issues, let alone so many. On our first Valentine's Day, he surprised me by making me a dinner of foods I could eat. I had never felt so loved and known through food.

For our wedding, a friend offered to make our cake and cupcakes. I gave her my list of no-no's, and she made the best gluten-free, sugar-free, dairy-free, soy-free—and too many other foods to list-free—cake I could have imagined. All this back in a world where food sensitivities and gluten-free eating were not so common, and fewer food options were available. This friend never complained but, even on her fixed income as a single mom, spent the time and money on all the special ingredients needed to make it happen. When people can see your boundaries and meet you in them, it is profoundly kind and generous.

Because of how I ate, all of my health issues were well under control. I had energy, clarity of mind, and the ability to live each day without being miserable. My husband was supportive. My friends were supportive. And I felt better than I had in my entire life.

After the dinner with my sister's missionary friends, when God gave me the grace to eat freely without getting sick, my eyes were opened wide to who I had always known God to be but had yet to experience—Healer. I'd always known God was our healer and that He could do anything. I'd known He was much bigger and more powerful than so many pastors and churches in my past believed Him to be. But to actually experience His radical healing in that one evening took me to new depths of faith that I had only dreamed of.

I knew I wasn't completely healed after that dinner, but God had clearly protected my body in the moment, giving me the grace to eat without getting sick. He had blessed the food to be good for my body, regardless of the nutrition facts or immune responses that could say otherwise. He heard my cries and answered me.

Once I realized I wasn't completely healed, I started asking the Lord for complete healing—something I had never even considered before. As I prayed about it, I knew He was going to heal me one day. One day, but I had no idea when.

My sister and I contended for it often in prayer, but I was also very content with my life, my health, and my diet as it was. Those food boundaries kept me healthy and on the straight and narrow as much as they kept my health issues in check. For the first time in my life, I had incredible self-control with food because I knew how awful I would feel if I didn't. In a weird way, I was thankful for it all.

Even still, life in those boundaries wasn't easy. I had to work hard to manage and plan for each day, for trips, and for social outings. My symptoms and health issues were well managed, but I still had occasional health flares that were nothing short of miserable. While I didn't need to be healed, I still wanted to be. I didn't need the freedom to eat anything and everything, but I wanted to be able to live my life without so much work and intentionality around food. I was content with the present circumstances, yet I yearned for something more. And now I knew that there was permission to desire that something more. In fact, it felt like the Lord was wanting me to accept that being fully healed was a good and righteous desire.

My prayers for healing were not ones of desperation or impatience. I knew, deep down in my bones, that one day He would heal me, and that's really all I needed to know. Life went on, and it was good, even in the midst of the restrictions.

After that one dinner with our friends, I gained faith to ask the Lord for help in different settings and situations. If we were invited over to someone's house for a meal, to a birthday party, or to another gathering that offered a slew of foods I knew I couldn't eat, I would ask the Lord what I should do. I'd ask Him what was most important in those moments.

At first, I assumed that He would always cover me and give me the grace to eat if I had a good enough reason to, but that wasn't actually His desire. Instead, He was teaching me how to lean in and ask for wisdom in each circumstance. It wasn't always the same answer, but He always answered. Because of that, I never felt like I was bound by my diet or health issues. When I needed grace to navigate the moment, it was there—preserving the value of the meal, the people, and the moment, while also preserving my body.

In the moment, if I didn't feel any clear direction, I considered what I had learned about His heart for food—all the good things it cultivates. I'd think about these things in direct tension with my health and dietary needs, never feeling like I had to sacrifice one for the other, but considering what was best. What was the Lord giving me peace about? When I invited the Lord into the process, He made a way. Sometimes I was able to find foods that worked within my boundaries and still enjoy the fellowship of others. Sometimes friends asked what my dietary needs were so they could make a meal that would accommodate me. Other times, I felt the Lord giving me the freedom to just eat and enjoy. Still other times He gave me specific instructions or strategies for what to eat or how much.

One day in particular, I went to a cookout with a new Bible study group I had joined. I didn't know many people and was still trying to get connected. The plan was to make and grill homemade pizzas, which were most definitely not on my list of safe foods.

It was only the second time I had ever sought to ask Jesus for help with a social engagement, the first being dinner with our missionary friends. As a backup, I brought some rice cakes and hummus for myself but planned to pray and consider eating if I had peace about it. After all, Jesus had told me to "eat" the last time I asked, so why would this be any different?

Once the pizzas were on the grill and I started praying about what to do, I didn't feel peace to eat freely. I didn't really know what God was saying at first. This pizza, without the Lord's help, was not only going to make me feel terrible but would trigger that awful celiac response, causing significant damage to my intestines and a host of other issues that would stem from it. I wanted to be very sure that, if I was going to eat, Jesus was going to cover me.

Not long before the pizza came off the grill, I finally felt the nudge of the Holy Spirit to just eat one slice and then to eat my rice cakes and hummus. Peace washed over my heart, all fear and uncertainty left and, while it wasn't what I was expecting, I knew it was the Lord's answer for that moment.

I only had one friend in the group at the time since I was still getting to know everyone. I shared with her what I was processing through and she prayed with me before we ate. Everyone dove into the pizzas, I into my one slice, and the conversations and fellowship flowed. After my one slice, I moved on to my rice cakes and hummus and felt like nothing skipped a beat. It wasn't awkward; no one really noticed. I was deeply satisfied by that one slice of pizza, feeling as though I had been able to partake of the meal with everyone while still being wise with what my body needed.

In His kindness, Jesus had protected my body once more, but He'd also asked me to honor my boundaries—albeit to a lesser degree—at the same time. I never got sick. Not one symptom came in the days following.

I could sit here and try to explain why Jesus said just one slice—in fact, I'd probably make a very good case of it—but the point wasn't for me to figure out His reasoning. It was for me to follow and trust, to bear witness to His goodness and kindness, and to be grateful in all things. The more I try to find the reasons He does what He does, the more I realize I am looking for a formula—one that will translate into other times and circumstances so I know what to do. But Jesus doesn't want us to function from a formula, He wants us to live in relationship with Him. He wants us to get to know His heart so that we can discern what wisdom is. And He wants to show us that He is always faithful.

The purpose of food is not so that we can have a relationship with food—whether a good one or a bad one—it's to enhance our relationship with Him.

As the months and years went on, I entered into numerous meals and circumstances that required hearing from Jesus to know what to do. Eventually, it became a way of life. I never hesitated to accept dinner invitations or stressed over celebrations and holidays. As sure as the ground was beneath my feet, I knew the Lord would give me a way through that didn't cost me my health. No matter the situation, it was never awkward because Jesus always gave me an answer that tended to the needs of all of us in the room. Many times, it wasn't just about me.

Interestingly, in three and a half years of invitations and events with food, Jesus never once told me to simply "not eat." Not once. I'm just now realizing this as I write, and I'm in awe at how profound it is. The Lord never once asked me to sit on the sidelines and observe as fellowship happened around food. He never expected me to be in a place where everyone else ate and I did not. He always made a way for what was important and, while food was not the focus, it was a unifying piece that He valued.

So my life went, living within boundaries while still experiencing freedom. I came to love this way of life and how close I felt to Jesus through it all. I still knew God would heal me, but I didn't think about it often. Life was good.

Then, one morning, everything flipped upside down when God spoke three potent words.

"You. Are. Healed."

chapter 13

freedom

I hadn't been actively praying for it, but it was so loud and clear in my mind that I jolted up in my chair. *Was that me? Or was that You, God?*

It couldn't have been me. I hadn't thought about or prayed about God healing me in months. It had been three and a half years since I first asked God to heal me, but in a weird way, I wasn't sure I really needed to be healed anymore. Life in my strict boundaries, with the freedom of Jesus to lead me out of them at times, was good; healing wasn't really necessary.

As I considered the voice—whether it was me or God—I came back to what I already knew deep down: clearly, this was God.

An overwhelming peace surrounded me and filled me. I could do nothing but sit in awe, full of worship but unable to speak or sing.

After an hour or so, His voice spoke again with the same crispness and clarity:

"It's because I love you."

At that, my entire body melted. My heart was completely undone. Who was I, that God would come in such extravagance and generosity, just because He loved me?

I had always believed that God would heal me because of some practical need—moving back overseas or living in circumstances with limited access to fresh foods, or maybe when my health issues got too bad. I never thought He would heal me just because He loved me.

For *four hours* I sat there, immersed in a thick invisible cloud of His presence, basking in His love. I wasn't even thinking about the practical changes this brought with it, or the freedom to eat whatever I wanted. It was such a holy moment that I never wanted it to end.

Gluten—especially in the form of wheat—was first on the list because, if I was truly healed, this would be the biggest test. For several days, I consumed wheat in a variety of forms, even unhealthy, processed forms. I never got sick. Then, one by one, I tried every other food that I would normally have had a significant reaction to. Days passed, and not one negative reaction. Every symptom of my former health issues was completely gone.

Testing would later confirm that my thyroid was also functioning normally for the first time in years. I was, in fact, healed. My husband and I were overjoyed. I could, after so many years, just *eat*.

After it was confirmed, it was time to go grocery shopping. *This is going to be so much fun*, I thought.

Or *so* I thought.

Once inside, I grabbed a cart and started down the aisles. So many options; I just walked and drooled for a while, taking it all in. Nothing was off limits. All the food choices I could dream of yet, after ten minutes, I hadn't placed one single thing in the cart. I walked up and down aisle after aisle considering what to buy but paralyzed from choosing. Then I realized...

I actually wanted my boundaries back.

Whaaaaat!?

This was so confusing. I thought it would be amazing, having this newfound freedom, but it was terrifying. My boundaries had been a safe place. They were restrictive, but they drew clear boundary lines that kept me eating good, clean foods. They kept me away from all the not-so-good foods—ones that I never used to have much self-control with.

I thought back to a friend in college who pretended to have health issues in order to force her to eat healthier. It seemed hilarious and absurd at the time. Now here I was, thinking much the same thing.

I stood there, lost in thought in the freezer section, when the Lord's voice came yet again.

"It's time to learn wisdom."

I immediately understood.

The past few years, I had learned to live in strict boundaries while still following the Lord into moments of freedom. Now, it was time to learn how to live in freedom, yet look to the Lord—rather than my boundaries—for the wisdom to guide me. Wisdom and freedom may seem antagonistic when it comes to food and diets but, in reality, they provide a beautiful and necessary balance to our lives.

Once the Lord spoke, I instantly had a vision of a young girl growing up in a house with her Father. He had built the house and everything in it to be safe for her. The four walls protected her from the outside world.

In that house, He taught her many things. He often took her outside the house to experience more of the world and, as He did, He held her hand, guided her, and protected her. She followed under His guard in those moments, enjoying new and exciting things before returning to the house with Him at the end of the day. Once there, she could let go of His hand to roam freely because she was back in a place of safety—her boundaries.

The young girl grew and matured. Each time the Father took her out of the house, He taught her more. He gave her more space to roam, not always needing to hold her hand, but still on guard to protect her from the things she could not yet navigate.

Then, one day, she was a young woman. The Father looked at her and said, "It's time to leave the house. These boundaries are no longer meant for you."

It came as a shock. The daughter was both thrilled with the possibilities of a new life—one with freedom to explore and live beyond what she had known—yet terrified to no longer have the protected space that had been so safe and set apart. She thought about her excursions with her Father, relishing the times when she got to be led by Him with such close protection and care. With this new freedom, would He be as near? Would it be as special?

No, she didn't want to leave. The world was uncertain and unsafe. This space had been good to her—comfortable and full of life—and she winced to think of saying goodbye to the walls around her.

The Father looked at the daughter, knowing all she was feeling. "If you stay, you will forsake all that I have prepared for you and all that I have prepared you for. This house, these boundaries, were only meant for a time, but now that time is over. It's time to step out and learn wisdom."

She considered His words with a bit of sorrow. "Will you still go with me?"

"I will always be there," He said with the greatest depth of love in His voice. "You will just need to remember to look to me when you need extra guidance."

With that, the vision ended.

I had grown accustomed to following Jesus out of my boundaries at times, asking for wisdom in each moment. With this vision I felt a supernatural empowerment from the Lord that the answers for how to navigate all things food related were now within me. Rather than letting the boundaries tell me how to eat or asking the Lord specifically what He was saying for every meal, outing, and circumstance, it was time to learn how to use my discernment and good judgement.

Good judgment, at this point, was completely different than my good judgment from several years ago. Why? Because Jesus had taken me on a journey where I had learned more about Him, His heart, His values, and food itself. Food was no longer just about health or enjoyment, but all the beautiful ways it reflects who He is and how He loves us.

After years of asking questions and embracing revelation from Him on the big things and little things, I learned my Father's ways. Soon, with enough practice, those ways became my ways—my own way of life. Learning to walk in freedom and wisdom was difficult at first. It took time for me to learn to live from such a heavenly mindset without the boundaries there to help. But, after enough practice, day to day wisdom became as simple as breathing.

Wisdom in freedom is full of tension—one that holds all the values that God created food for in balance. There will be moments and seasons when certain values will be more important than others—more dominant—but the other values still remain. They are not cast off. All things have a time and season, and wisdom seamlessly guides us through them all.

chapter 14

seasons

Every good thing has value in the right season. But every good thing can also become a stumbling block when we force it into the wrong season, the wrong setting, or the wrong circumstance. This is why we can't make blanket statements or generalizations about nutrition. It's why our personal experience with food, diets, or health issues won't translate to someone else's. It's why what's worked in the past may not work in the present.

Trying to hold on to answers that are not right for us or the season we're in can be like forcing a square peg through a round hole. It doesn't fit well without a lot of force and frustration.

As such, it's important we seek to know the season we're in when we consider how to eat. This will keep us from setting unhealthy goals, measuring ourselves against wrong standards, and taking on burdens that the Lord never intended for us to carry. Instead, when we understand the season we are in, we can better discern what steps to take, what prayers to pray, when to wait on the Lord, and when to act.

Twelve years ago, I found answers for my health issues through a specific type of food sensitivity test and a strict gluten-free diet. I researched, studied, and learned all that I could in relation to these things so that I could implement them into my work with patients. In fact, these were the very things that propelled me into private practice.

Everywhere I looked, I saw people with health issues that would most certainly be remedied by this test and implementing the diet changes that go along with it. I became a broken record advocating for it. Often, I was right. Many patients, family, and friends saw tremendous health improvements. But that wasn't always the story that unfolded.

My sister, Lonni, for example, was dealing with some pretty significant stomach issues that I was convinced would be remedied by this protocol. She wasn't as convinced, but eventually she decided to go for it because she was so miserable. After a week of feeling worse, suddenly her symptoms abated, and her health improved tremendously. All the improvements I had hoped to see were there, yet she was cranky and not super stoked about it.

This new, personalized way of eating was manageable, but it was also very extreme for her. It never sat well with her emotionally—it never gave her peace or a sense of hope. Rather, it felt burdensome and discouraging.

Eventually she decided it was no longer for her and gradually went back to her old ways of eating. Once she was able to get past feeling as though she had failed and to let go of what she thought she "should" be doing, she remembered the Holy Spirit had nudged her *not* to do this protocol back before she ever started. Yet she had pushed that nudge, that invitation to trust and wait for the right step, aside. In exchange, she picked up my solutions—at my urging—and all the heavy burdens that came with it. Hope drained out of her and a sense of heavy, restrictive responsibility set in.

Once she went back to her normal way of eating, her symptoms returned. Reason would say that these dietary changes were what she needed to do to heal, because clearly they helped, but that wasn't the truth. Her symptoms may have returned with her dietary departure, but so did her peace. As she remembered hearing the Lord's voice all those weeks before, nudging her not to do the protocol in the first place, she felt hopeful. Even though *this* wasn't the answer, an answer would surely come.

What can seem like a divine answer to one person, full of life and hope, can be a heavy burden to someone else, stealing life and hope. It took me years to realize that not everyone needed *my* answers. They needed their own. What was good for me in my season wasn't always good and right for other people in their seasons.

The Lord healed Lonni a few years later, after a long journey of emotional healing and restoring hope to her spirit. It was both a gradual healing through various means over time and then a final instant healing that eradicated the issue once and for all. Food sensitivities were never intended to be a part of her journey, but they were meant to be a part of mine.

It took me years to understand this in my practice with my patients. The answers that seem to fit by knowledge and research alone need to be measured against the person, their life, their season, their circumstances, as well as the Holy Spirit. I didn't just need head knowledge, I needed discernment to see the person as a whole. I needed discernment to know what tools, what information, and what advice would be most beneficial. What, of my library of knowledge and resources, was the Lord highlighting for *them*?

This seems like a tall order, but it's not. It simply takes stepping back and seeing the bigger picture before zooming in to figure out what's really needed. I had to learn to do this for my patients, but I am also learning how to help my patients do this for themselves. Each of us knows our own body, our own heart, our season, and our capacity better than anyone else. As much as I can offer insight and advice to a patient, they have to determine if it is right for them, to discern what things are wise to take and pursue, and to dismiss those that aren't. I use my best discernment, but they also need to use theirs.

It's easy to assume that we know what we need to pursue, especially if our health is at stake. We are in no short supply of health information, opinions, and testimonials—all of which can muffle our understanding of who we are and what it is that we truly need. We are surrounded by false standards of what we think we need to achieve, never realizing that those standards are not always ours to own.

The good news is that Jesus knows us better than we know ourselves. If we step back, tune into His presence around us, and simply ask, He will help us find the right steps and the right answers in time. We can't follow Jesus on a road that we create for ourselves because He isn't there. We can't follow Him on a road intended for someone else because He isn't there either. We have to follow Him where He leads us, the path He has marked out for us alone. That path will change as seasons and circumstances change, but it is the path where the Lord's blessing will flow.

We may not always have a clear course set before us, so it's okay to try things out—taking steps forward, and then stepping back to reevaluate and recalibrate. Remember, it is often a journey Jesus is leading us on rather than a clear and concise step or a quick solution. He is not in a hurry with us because there is more at stake in our hearts and lives than we realize through the process.

Solomon himself talked about the times and seasons of life being ever changing.

> "a time to be born and a time to die,
> a time to plant and a time to uproot…
> a time to tear down and a time to build,
> a time to weep and a time to laugh,
> a time to mourn and a time to dance…
> a time to embrace and a time to refrain,
> a time to search and a time to give up,
> a time to keep and a time to throw away,
> a time to tear and a time to mend,
> a time to be silent and a time to speak,
> a time to love and a time to hate,
> a time for war and a time for peace."
> ECCLESIASTES 3:2-8

Different seasons and different circumstances will inevitably be marked with different needs. If we don't first survey and acknowledge the season of life we are living in, we can easily trip ourselves up by expecting too much or too little of ourselves as a result. But if we understand those seasons and give value to them, we will find hope and wisdom that will both bless our bodies and revive our hearts.

To expound a little more on Solomon's words, think about some different scenarios. Wisdom for our health in a time of war or great turmoil—think World War II or the Great Depression—will look different from wisdom for our health in peacetime. It will look different in seasons of abundance—with extra time, resources, and emotional capacity—versus seasons of limited capacity—perhaps more emotionally charged or busier seasons, with more constraints. Wisdom will be different in a time of health crisis, where healing is needed, versus a time of good health.

Within these seasons are times for different things. There is a time for more dietary boundaries and a time for more freedom. A time to embrace change and a time to refrain. A time to celebrate more and worry less. A time to search out answers and a time to wait and trust. A time for more discipline and a time for more grace.

Like a river, wisdom ebbs and flows, changing with every season and every circumstance both big and small. It's not hard to find wisdom, we just need to remember to look for her. She is always there to show us the way. She is alive and ever changing—dynamic, not static.

Food isn't meant to be the focus in each season in life. In fact, it rarely is meant to be the absolute focus at all. Food is an expression of something bigger, whether it is community, celebration, covenant, generosity, faith, enjoyment, grieving, healing, growing, or rest—or anything else beyond that. The heartbeat of it all, the focus of the moments and seasons, is not food but what is happening around it. Food is very much a part of those seasons, sometimes more dominant a part than other times, but it's not the point of it.

Don't get lost in the diets. Get lost in the heart of the Father. Everything flows from there. This is where we feel most satisfied and most capable, because this is where our grace is. It is where we will feel most content, most hopeful and most at rest within our spirits. This is where health and healing are found.

Let's talk more about constraints. Some constraints are fixed things that we cannot change, others are things we can change but feel powerless or unmotivated to. Identifying and acknowledging them will help us discern how to move forward victoriously. Lay all of those challenges before the Lord, and ask Him for help and wisdom, for creative solutions to know how to navigate them. We may not be able to change some circumstances, but the Lord is good to show us what we can do within them.

Unrecognized constraints can produce a lot of shame and guilt. When we do not acknowledge them, we tend to think it's our fault that we're failing. Some people can become a victim of their limitations—discouraged, hopeless, and possibly resentful. Jesus wants to come into those places, to overwhelm us with supernatural help and hope tailored specifically to us in the midst of them.

I've seen picky eaters find an abundance of foods they love; people who hate to cook develop a passion for food prep in simple, realistic ways. I've seen people on a fixed income thrive in their health, even on non-organic foods, by simply being faithful with what they have. I've watched Jesus give permission not to worry about people's food choices in light of other life events, but then bring them back to it later when their hearts are healthy and their lives conducive. There simply is no limit to how God can answer you and lead you through the seasons.

chapter 15

opposition

A year after God healed me, I started feeling poorly again. It was gradual at first—a mild symptom here, another symptom there. But, before I knew it, I was snowballing back towards my old health issues. I didn't understand it, but I couldn't ignore it. God had healed me, this I knew. Maybe this was a new health issue, or perhaps something different altogether, but I needed answers.

When your body feels at war with itself, you become desperate for solutions. I was desperate. I had learned to love my freedom, by this point, and thought I had done well learning wisdom in what and how I ate. Even still, it didn't seem to matter. My body was breaking all over again.

After grieving the loss of my healing, I decided it was time to buck up and find some strict boundaries again. I pulled all the common food triggers out of my diet, had some blood work done and, based on the test results, I omitted a handful of other foods that were triggering my immune system. It worked; I felt great. All those awful symptoms went away, and I was back to feeling healthy—at least physically healthy. Inside, however, my spirit withered.

When I began the restrictive way of eating the first time around all those years ago, it felt good and life giving. I knew it was from the Lord, an answer to many of my cries for help. This time, however, it felt like defeat. I felt bound. My heart didn't feel hopeful or at peace, but sorrowful and discouraged. It didn't feel right or good, but I didn't know what else to do.

About a month into the new boundaries, Lonni came over for lunch. She saw my gluten-free bread and all the specialty foods in my fridge, and she was puzzled. I told her about changing my diet again and all the symptoms that had returned. I told her how I didn't like it, but changing my diet made me feel better. It didn't matter what I said, she was indignant at the idea of me going backwards.

"When Jesus healed you, He healed you," she said. "Why are you allowing yourself to go back to a place that He already delivered you from?"

I didn't have a great answer. If it worked and I felt better, why wouldn't I?

Over the next week, I couldn't get Lonni's voice out of my head. I agreed with her wholeheartedly; there was just no way to reconcile the truth of it to what I was experiencing.

A week later, I went to the park with a former patient and her son. Rachel and I had become friends through her health journey and kept in touch every so often once she stopped being a patient.

Rachel and her toddler-aged son had a lot of health issues. For years we worked through layer after layer of issues, addressing them with ever-changing dietary protocols and supplements. With each change, things would mildly improve, and a few weeks later they would get worse again in some other way. It was a never-ending cycle that we couldn't get past. Eventually Rachel and her son each had a list of ten or fifteen foods they could safely eat without having a severe reaction—mind you that each of their lists was different from the other.

Rachel went to several additional practitioners after working with me, experiencing much the same outcome each time. One step forward, one step back. Their food lists changed at times, but it never grew to more than a handful of foods.

Back to the day at the park. It was perfect weather, and we found a nice picnic table to sprawl out at. She pulled out their lunches, laying one food item after another on the table for her son to choose from. I'm sure she knew I was looking at what they were eating, and she knew how shocked I would be, but she didn't say anything. She ate, he ate, and I sat there dumbfounded. Not one food item in those meals had been on their safe list of foods for years. Most of the foods had been huge triggers for them, even since before I started working with them; but here they were, eating as free as birds and clearly loving the ability to do so. Before I could get the words out of my mouth to ask, Rachel began to share.

In the past year, they had sought the help from other holistic practitioners. As a result, they had added numerous diets, protocols, and therapies onto what they were already doing. Over time, the rules and protocols became too much. She felt like they were putting her and her son in some sort of bondage that was heavy and hard to manage. Through that year of struggle, God began teaching her to trust Him more with their health. She had always been a proficient researcher on Google and through various books to learn more about health and nutrition, desperate to find answers. As her faith began to grow, she committed to stop the constant researching and striving. In doing so, her spirit felt free, but the health issues persisted. She continued working with those health care practitioners, but nothing they offered seemed to provide solutions.

Then came an invitation for Rachel and her son to go on a day excursion with some friends. Normally this would have been a firm "no," as full day outings weren't manageable with each of their strict dietary needs. This time, however, rather than saying no, she felt a deep conviction from the Lord that this was no longer okay. Food wasn't allowed to rule their lives and it was time to start believing Jesus for His ability to heal, even before that healing came.

So, in faith, she prayed, and they went. They ate food with complete freedom and enjoyed the day to the fullest. At the end of the day, not one symptom. The next day, they still felt great. It was a complete miracle and the day that changed everything. Rachel was determined to start eating in faith, and to let go of all the insane food boundaries they had been living in for years. With this, food stopped being their enemy. Their bodies could now receive it as a blessing, no longer causing the problematic symptoms they had faced for so long.

I sat and listened to Rachel, very aware that God was speaking something similar to me. At some point in the previous year, I had adopted the belief that food was my enemy. If I felt sick, food was to blame. Never mind that I had seen and learned the goodness of God through food; I had somehow forgotten. I hadn't thought to ask God for answers to my health dilemma; I just sought them out on my own, assuming they were the same answers as last time.

A deep conviction pierced my heart through Rachel's story. I had a choice to view food as a gift once more; to eat in faith; to let go of trying to fix myself in my own strength. So I went to the grocery store, purchased all the foods I had been avoiding, and went home to eat. I made my sandwich—intentionally putting every ingredient I could think of in it that I had been avoiding. Once that glorious lunch was made, I sat down, thanked God, and ate. As I did, it was as though my heart came back to life.

No symptoms followed that meal, nor any of the ones to come in the following days. The food had indeed blessed my body to nourish it and I was, yet again, undone by the goodness of God. The Lord restored my faith and my health that day. I was still healed; I had just allowed myself to be convinced that I wasn't. It's important to know when to stand in faith for what we know to be true, whatever that truth is, and not let the enemy or circumstances convince us otherwise.

That was not the last time I faced a health crisis where some, or all of those old symptoms, or new symptoms started to creep in. Heidi Baker wrote in her book Reckless Devotion, "Satan is trying to destroy your destiny, God's temple. If he can't use sin, he will use sickness or exhaustion. So, we have to fight."

The way we fight is by looking at Jesus.

I couldn't list all the times my health came under fire over the next several years if I tried. There are simply too many to recall. But every time something flared up, I found that it wasn't wise to lean on old answers if that wasn't where Jesus and discernment were leading me. Old answers tend to produce formulas, and formulas produce rules; rules do not impart life. Rules don't know us and our circumstances; they can't rescue or deliver us. They can't breathe life into our spirits. **But Jesus can.**

Instead, I've learned to ask Jesus for help; to ask Him, "What is this?" and, "What should I do?"

If we have to fight for our health at times, we need to be clear about two things: what it is that we are really up against, and how the Lord is leading us to navigate it. We need wisdom in times of crisis just like we need wisdom in times of good health and abundance, just like we need wisdom in seasons of boundaries as well as seasons of freedom.

> "If any of you lacks wisdom, he should ask God, who gives generously to all without finding fault, and it will be given to him. But when he asks, he must believe and not doubt, because he who doubts is like a wave of the sea, blown and tossed by the wind."
>
> JAMES 1:5-6

Sometimes we come to Jesus hoping for a crumb of wisdom, just enough to give us answers. But He doesn't give us crumbs. He isn't the God of "just enough." He is the God of abundance, the God who gives wisdom *generously*, as the book of James states.

Our job is to ask and then to believe Him when He speaks. The enemy would love nothing more than to convince us that we are the ones responsible to find our own answers and fix ourselves. But that's a lie. If we don't believe He will help us, it will be hard to hear Him past all the other noise around us and within us. He won't force Himself on us. He wants us to choose to listen, and that means trusting that He will answer.

The Lord never intends to hide wisdom so that we cannot find her. On the contrary, Solomon declares that wisdom calls out to us. She longs to be found. She raises her voice to be heard. She stands at the doors of our coming and going, hoping that we will pay attention and heed her.

> "Does not wisdom call out? Does not understanding raise her voice? On the heights along the way, where the paths meet, she takes her stand; besides the gates leading into the city, at the entrances, she cries aloud: 'To you, O men, I call out; I raise my voice to all mankind."
>
> PROVERBS 8:1-4

Wisdom calls out to each of us and to all of mankind. If we don't know what it is, it's simply because we didn't ask, we didn't believe, or because we are still waiting and Jesus is going to pour it out soon.

It's important to recognize that there is no endpoint for our health journey. That's not to say there isn't victory; that there isn't healing from health issues and restoration of good health; that there isn't a way of eating that is right for you in the season you are in to get you where you need to go. But we will never "arrive" with regard to our health—at least not until we get to heaven. There will always be new challenges and new seasons. As long as we are on earth, living in bodies that age, wear out, break, and change, our health will endure challenges. We will need wisdom again and again and again. The good news is that wisdom flows freely from Jesus and will always be given to those who seek it.

Not one of us is without hope for our health. Wisdom is ours for the taking if we want it—true wisdom that brings life, hope, and healing. Wisdom that is not hard, heavy, or confusing.

Look for her in each step you take, in each decision you make.

Whether you need healing or to live a healthy life in a world that feels too unhealthy to manage, she is for you. Search for wisdom in the midst of all the options in front of you, and the Lord will make her known. Jesus, the One who makes a road in the wilderness and streams in a desert, is capable of so much more than we can imagine. He can—and *will*—guide you and do impossible things for you if you allow Him to, simply because He loves you.

chapter 16

the fruit

I'm often asked, "How do you know if it's wisdom? How do you know if you are actually hearing God's voice or sensing His leading? If you are discerning right and making good choices in His eyes?"

Simply put, we will know the source of something by the fruit it produces. Wisdom from the Spirit of God will produce fruit of the Spirit.

> "But the wisdom that comes from heaven is first of all pure; then peace-loving, considerate, submissive, full of mercy and *good fruit*, impartial and sincere. Peacemakers who sow in peace raise a harvest of righteousness."
> JAMES 3:17-18 (emphasis mine)

So here we have the test of wisdom: Does it feel pure? Does it produce peace? Is it considerate of others and humble in heart? Does it carry mercy? Is it impartial to the opinion of others? Is it sincere? And finally, does it produce good fruit in your life and in the lives of those around you? We can ask these things regarding our diet, our health journey, and our way of eating to know if we are actually walking in step with the Lord in this part of our lives.

Consider how Jesus talks about wisdom from the world verses wisdom from the Father:

> "For John the Baptist came neither eating bread nor drinking wine, and you say, 'He has a demon.' The Son of Man came eating and drinking, and they say, 'Here is a glutton and a drunkard, a friend of tax collectors and "sinners!"' But *wisdom is proved right by her children.*"
>
> LUKE 7:33-35 (emphasis mine)

The world of nutrition is much like these verses—often contradicting itself, disputing any diet or decision for something thought to be better. Jesus faced religious people that had developed formulas for holiness, but their formulas had nothing solid to stand on. The religious Jews were constantly contradicting themselves because wisdom from heaven operated in a way that they simply couldn't understand or replicate.

Our bent, as humans, is to figure things out. "How to" books, blogs, videos, and articles permeate our culture, most of which say opposing things. Jesus speaks to this pursuit of wisdom, and essentially says that wisdom is not measured by the method—how you eat or what you do—it's measured by what it produces. True wisdom is "proved right by her children." In other words, true wisdom cultivates things that are full of life.

Jesus proves that two different ways of life, ways that seem completely contradictory to one another, can both be wisdom. John the Baptist did not eat bread or drink wine, and he was criticized. It didn't seem right to the religious sect because it didn't fit their laws or understanding. Likewise, Jesus Himself was criticized for doing just the opposite. He came eating and drinking and was then labeled a glutton and drunkard.

The world cannot understand godly wisdom and will often criticize what they can't understand. Rules and laws, diets and formulas are all the world knows apart from Jesus. But wisdom does not hinge on these things. It hinges on the Spirit of God fueling us and informing us, and it is proved right by the fruit of what comes of it. All the worldly knowledge we have is still valuable, as I have said many times before; but all the information in the world without the breath of God fueling us is hollow and powerless.

Anything from the Spirit of God is intended to bear good fruit. Initially you might think this fruit is the physical health of a person. Does it accomplish good things for their physical body? But, if you have been paying attention thus far, you will quickly figure out that wisdom is not measured by a physical outcome alone. If we physically transform but inwardly become frustrated, anxious, discouraged, sad, sorrowful, fearful, self-focused, or all-consumed, then the fruit is rotten. It doesn't breed more life; it takes life. That tells us we haven't yet found the wisdom we need.

Relationship with Jesus is the key to wisdom. It is the reason formulas will never be enough for us. It's the reason a diet alone, information alone, cannot fully fix or satisfy. We were created to be in relationship with Him—it is from this place that we learn and discover wisdom for every moment and season of life.

If you aren't sure if you are living in wisdom, look at the fruit. Whatever form wisdom takes, it will bear good fruit.

One thing I have found to be true time and time again is that Jesus is very spiritual but also wildly practical. He loves to help us with practical things, things we often neglect to ask for help with.

For example, I often ask the Lord to bless my body to crave what it needs—foods that will be good for it, life giving, and enjoyable. He has always answered. I have patients that pray when they go grocery shopping for new ideas and new foods that fit in their boundaries and budget for that season. I have other patients who hate meal prep or cooking at home, and they have prayed for Jesus to help them enjoy what they formerly despised. Each of these examples are ones where God faithfully answered each person, and continues to. Each is a story I could tell that would leave you in awe of how God answered because, although His response was practical, it was still profoundly supernatural.

Jesus cares about the little practical things in our lives and will equip us with the practical tools we need. I encourage you to test Him in this and see how He will come through for you.

Many people have been deceived to think that they are walking in wisdom through staunch self-discipline and negative mindsets about food, but there is nothing redemptive about that. A truly healthy person sees food beyond the parameters of physical health alone, from a heavenly perspective. Let's celebrate the freedom Jesus gives us to enjoy food and honor His charge to steward it well. Food is temporary, but the fruit that it cultivates in us and around us is eternal.

PART THREE
barriers to health

chapter 17

divine health

In the middle of the Garden of Eden stood the tree of life. At the beginning of creation, man was given direct access to it and all the fruit it produced—fruit that would give them, and their physical bodies, life everlasting. We were never created to eventually wear out and die but rather to live. When Adam and Eve sinned by eating of the tree of the knowledge of good and evil, they were banished from the Garden of Eden and from the tree of life itself.

> "And the Lord God said, 'The man has become like one of us, knowing good and evil. He must not be allowed to reach out his hand and take also from the tree of life and eat, and live forever.'"
> GENESIS 3:22

Man would no longer live forever. This is the moment where human bodies became mortal, where we no longer had access to the life-giving fruit that would sustain our bodies forever. Sickness and disease, aging, and physical ailments entered into the world. Man was driven out of the Garden of Eden, the very place where the Lord had walked with man and lived among them. And so, not only did our physical bodies become mortal, but we became disconnected from God's very presence as well.

It's not how God designed it—infirmities, disease, death, or disconnection from Him—but when sin entered in the world, so did these challenges. Yet, in the great mercy of God, He planned redemption from the beginning.

All that Satan accomplished with Adam and Eve, Jesus soon overcame on the cross. When Jesus suffered, died, and rose from the grave, resurrection life entered the world. We are given the Holy Spirit to live within us—connecting us back to the Father and our Savior, restoring our intimate relationship with Him. Everything evil, everything painful, everything hopeless could now be redeemed into something beautiful. There is no sickness that cannot be healed, no disease that cannot be overcome, and the reality of death in this world only means a wonderful eternity with Jesus in a place where sickness and disease do not exist. Evil no longer wins in our lives or our health; that is, unless we allow it to.

Jesus warned us before He was crucified, saying,

> **"I have told you these things, so that in me you may have peace. In this world you will have trouble. But take heart! I have overcome the world."**
> JOHN 16:33

For many of us, those troubles have included some sort of health struggle—be it big or small. We ought not be surprised when we face health challenges. Instead, we can anchor into these two promises: with Jesus, there is peace in the midst of the storm, and He *will* overcome. Redemption is always a part of our story.

> **"...He took up our infirmities and carried our diseases"**
> MATTHEW 8:17

In this imperfect world, our bodies will age, and we may face health challenges along the way. But with Jesus, we will always find victory. He will do infinitely more for us than the trials attempt to take away.

> "Praise the Lord, O my soul, and forget not all His benefits—who forgives all your sins and heals all your diseases, who redeems your life from the pit and crowns you with love and compassion, who satisfies your desires with good things so that your youth is renewed like the eagles."
>
> PSALM 103:2-5

All throughout scripture we find promises like this, declaring the healing and redemptive nature of our Savior. It's who He is. As such, there is far more hope for us than we often realize, and we need to choose to anchor into that hope every day of our lives.

Jesus, what is this?

It's the question I have learned to ask time and time again when my health spirals, when physical challenges arise. My former instincts were to turn straight to nutrition and supplements and, if needed, to lab tests in order to find my answers.

Several years ago, I was struggling with severe gastrointestinal upset for weeks. As a functional nutrition expert, I was quick to diagnose myself, tweak my diet, and beeline for my over-sized supplement drawer to treat it and find relief. On this particular day, I found myself rummaging through that supplement drawer when the Holy Spirit's conviction landed on my heart like a brick.

"Stop."

It was calm and clear, and seemed to breathe a peaceful stillness into my spirit that was completely opposite to the desperation and striving I had been presently immersed in. That one word was all I heard, but the conviction of it spoke volumes. It was time to stop always trying to figure things out, to stop attempting to diagnose and fix myself with every ailment that came my way.

Not long before this day, my husband had challenged me in much the same way. "Why do you always have to figure it out?" I was constantly telling him how poorly I felt, what I thought was causing it, and what I needed to do to fix myself. I'd change my diet, take some supplements and eventually get better, but soon enough another ailment would creep in. Over and over Nathan would listen to my diagnostic process, but He was growing quite annoyed by it all.

"Why don't you try not to focus on it so much?" he'd say.

How do you ignore feeling so poorly? I thought. *Why wouldn't I try to figure it out so I could feel better? It's what I was trained to do. Isn't it a gift that I have so much knowledge to know what to do?*

I thought Nathan was being critical and lacking compassion. That is, until the Holy Spirit came in and convicted me of this very same thing. I had become the very personification of striving. I knew how to step back and pray over the bigger, more significant health flares, but the smaller ones, the annoying ones, the constant ones, I just assumed responsibility for myself.

With the conviction of the Lord, I began to see how all my striving was only getting me so far. I was trapped in an endless cycle because I never stepped back to gain discernment from the Lord for what was going on with my body before turning to my knowledge and resources to get answers. Without leaning on the Lord for understanding, without stepping back to pray for discernment, I was caught up in a whirlwind of noise and distraction. It wasn't peaceful or hopeful, and it consumed my focus, my finances, and my time.

In the quest for answers, we can easily make a lot of assumptions—it must be the food I'm eating, must be stress, must be this or that. Or we can presume to know what we need—diet changes, supplements, medications, etc. While these are all legitimate possibilities, there may be something more we need to see and understand first, something beyond face value. There may be other reasons our health is struggling: spiritual barriers such as sin, afflictions from the enemy, or disconnection from God. There could be emotional barriers or perhaps a significant purpose for which God is allowing us to be tested.

After the Holy Spirit's intervention that day, this one question became my anchor:

Jesus, what is this?

I have faced many health challenges and trials over the years for which I found wisdom in dietary and supplemental changes, but I have also faced challenges and trials that were completely unrelated to my diet. Sometimes it was spiritual, sometimes it was nutritional, sometimes it was emotional, and sometimes it was a combination of various things.

I've learned to trust the Lord's story over my own expectations because I can be confident in His faithfulness over my ability to figure it all out. With this, I have peace even when I don't *feel* okay because with Jesus, I know that I am okay. He will lead me to the right answers in time.

Once I discern what it is that I am up against, I then look for wisdom regarding how to move forward:

Jesus, what are You saying? What are you asking me to do?

Discerning wisdom, what the right next steps are, hinges on us knowing where the battle truly lies. Is it flesh? Is it spirit? Is it emotions? Is it a trial sent to test us?

Part Three of this book will seek to expound on some of these barriers to health and potential purposes for the struggle. While not exhaustive in its contents, it will hopefully increase your awareness, giving you more discernment when you need answers.

No matter how obvious it may seem, only Jesus knows the full story of what's happening and why. If we chase what seems obvious before we pause to ask for His insight, we might very well be chasing a squirrel down a never-ending rabbit hole where our answers do not fully exist. But if we take time to seek Jesus for insight and understanding, He will lead us down the right path where life-giving answers can always be found.

Our goal is not to pick apart our lives and over-analyze them. Rather, we simply need to first understand what it is that we're up against and why. When do we take a health issue at face value, and when do we look deeper?

We might discern right away that there is something deeper going on, but it may take some time after seeking the Lord to gain revelation as to what that something deeper is. Be patient but be persistent in prayer until the understanding comes. Once it does, you can better discern how to respond more effectively—knowing more acutely what to focus on and what to let go of. Search out the knowledge and practical tools you truly need versus all the information out there you could latch onto.

> **"For the Lord gives wisdom,**
> **And from His mouth comes knowledge**
> **and understanding.**
> **he holds victory in store for the upright,**
> **he is a shield for those whose walk is blameless,**
> **For he guards the course of the just, and protects the**
> **way of his faithful ones."**
>
> PROVERBS 2:6-8

chapter 18

sin & disconnection

When I was 22, God had very clearly put before me the opportunity to be a missionary in Malawi. I was excited about it, and He confirmed multiple times that it was the right step. Yet, in the following months, the reality of being a young missionary overseas started to overwhelm me. I questioned my decision and the radical encounter I'd had with Jesus when He called me to go and, as a result, decided to sweep things under the rug for a time. I continually put off turning in my application or doing anything to make it happen and continued on with my life as though it wasn't there.

My life was good, I loved my friends, and I didn't want to let go of it all. I was like Jonah, running the opposite direction, trying to be satisfied with being less than who I knew God had made me to be, and with doing less than I knew He had prepared for me to do.

As weeks passed, my life became less and less comfortable. Within the course of two months I was in three car wrecks that were all my fault. The first was on my way to my college class one morning. The second was in the rental car I was driving while my car was being repaired. The third collision happened as soon as my car was repaired, and the first day I was back driving it. Not fun.

In addition to the car wrecks, I managed to get three traffic tickets within those same two months. The first was a bother, but I could pay a fine and do a driving course to get it removed from my record. The second ticket meant my only option to keep it off my record was to pay the fine and spend a year on probation. This meant I couldn't get another ticket for a year in order to get the ticket to stay off of my record. When I got the third traffic ticket a few months later, I burst into tears. Another hefty fine on my already empty wallet, and both the second and third tickets went on my record for the next several years in addition to the two car wrecks.

A week later I became severely sick with what seemed like the flu. Getting sick, at that point in my life, was rare and especially rarer that I would have a high fever for two weeks without relent. Nothing helped. No medicine could reduce my fever, and my body seemed incapable of getting better.

I was undone. I called my sister in tears, agonizing over what on earth was happening to me and to my life. She listened quietly and was very slow to respond. It was evident that she felt the Lord was saying something, but I sensed her hesitation to share it, concerned that it might offend me.

Finally, she spoke.

"Laura, I don't really know how to say this."

Long pause.

"All I hear God saying is that He is disciplining you."

Another long pause.

I took in those words, and they went deep. Had they not been from the Holy Spirit Himself, I might have been offended—but I wasn't. It actually brought joy and vitality back into me, like a life-giving arrow to my soul. My life had truly become one of chaos—not because I was a victim of life's cruel circumstances like I thought, but because I was delaying and ignoring the very thing God had invited me to do. I had given Him my "yes" and then taken it back. In doing so, I had cut myself off from my source of life.

Those words broke me open, and yet they made me fall in love with Jesus all the more. Fear had caused me to lose sight of the reality that being a missionary was actually what my heart wanted, deep down. I was afraid of everything I had to let go of and had settled for a life of comfort rather than one of faith. Fear has a way of numbing our hearts to the point where we don't even realize we are not following the Lord's leading anymore.

When God confronted me through my sister, it wasn't about the work He'd called me to; it was about Him and me. I had taken my eyes off of Him, and so my heart and health followed.

I repented almost immediately and decided it was time to pursue the work I was neglecting. I finished my application and started taking steps toward life overseas. Sure enough, the cycle of catastrophes stopped at that point, with no more sickness.

A year later, I was living in Mzuzu, Malawi. For two years, I ran the foodservice operations of our childcare program that grew from fifteen to over four hundred meals each day. I got to know each of the young children that came into our care, watching them transform from sickly, withdrawn orphans into vivacious healthy children.

Those two years awakened a part of me that I didn't know existed. Without the comforts of my previous life in America, I rose to challenges I would have run away from before and discovered I was capable of so much more than I thought. It opened my eyes to the world beyond first-world luxuries—to the vast disparities between different walks of life. And in it all, it was the first time I actually found myself in love with Jesus. It was the time when His word became my source of life.

I loved my two years in Malawi. They weren't easy, but nothing worthwhile ever is. When I came back to the U.S. in 2008, I was a completely different person. The entire trajectory of my life shifted after that and, twelve years later, I still see how those two years were essential to everything that has followed since.

Where would I have ended up, had God not stepped in and gotten my attention so abruptly all those years ago by letting circumstances go crazy and my health fall apart? Thank you, Jesus, for letting my life break for a time so that I could be made whole.

> "I know, O Lord, that your laws are righteous, and in faithfulness you have afflicted me."
> PSALM 119:75

It's easy to blame food, genetics, or even God Himself when we are the victim of a broken body, but the reality might be that we have cut ourselves off from His protection and blessing somewhere down the road when we partnered with sin.

Until sin is confessed, it plagues us like a cancer. It can wreak havoc on our spirits, our minds, and our physical bodies. It hides in the shadows, convincing us that it's not that big of a deal, that it's not really sin, that it's more shameful to expose it than to just let it stay hidden and unknown. The truth is, once sin is allowed into the light to be seen, and we humble ourselves in repentance before our gracious Father, every ounce is then fully covered by the blood of Jesus. Forgiveness comes in an instant, restoring us completely in the Father's love. Confessed sin ceases to have power over us or hold any remnant of authority in our lives.

> "Some became fools through their rebellious ways and **suffered affliction because of their iniquities.** They loathed all food and drew near the gates of death.
>
> Then they cried to the Lord in their trouble, and he saved them from their distress. He sent forth his word and healed them; he rescued them from the grave.
>
> Let them give thanks to the Lord for his unfailing love and his wonderful deeds for men. Let them sacrifice thank offerings and tell of his works with songs of joy."
> PSALM 107:17-20 (emphasis mine)

Some of us need to consider that our health may be suffering as a result of our choices—choices that go against what the Lord is saying, choices that go against what is good and right and holy.

> "And if the Spirit of him who raised Jesus from the dead is living in you, he who raised Christ from the dead will also give life to your mortal bodies through His Spirit, who lives in you...For if you live according to the sinful nature, you will die; but if by the Spirit you put to death the misdeeds of the body, you will live, because those who are led by the Spirit of God are the sons of God."
>
> ROMANS 8:11,13

Sin breaks down our bodies and breeds death. It is contrary to the Spirit of God that gives life. Ultimately, if we are choosing sin—whether it is being disobedient to something God spoke or an ungodly act that you know is contrary to righteousness—it will suffocate the life-giving Spirit of God within us, leaving us more vulnerable to sickness and disease.

Praise God when our bodies break so our sin can be exposed. Better to be sick for a time and made right with God, than never to be sick but have a festering soul. The beautiful reality in all of this is that Jesus is right there, waiting for us to cry out to Him. His promise is certain: He will forgive us, heal us, and restore us.

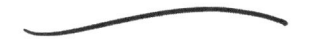

How do you know if your health issues stem from unconfessed sin? That revelation comes from God alone, and it starts with inquiring of Him for discernment. It wasn't until my world seemed to be imploding on me that I finally cried out to understand why. At the time, I didn't think to ask God for insight, but my sister did. I have her to thank for seeking God's insight, but Him to thank even more for giving it.

As I have grown and matured in my walk with Jesus, I am much more aware of times when I sin against Him. It grieves my spirit deeply, and I yearn to know when it happens so I can be quick to repent. It's not the fear of being sick that motivates me now, or the troubles sin can bring with it. It's because I want nothing to come between me and Jesus. I want to be like Him in every way, living my life under the authority of truth.

Sin is obvious to the one who is sinning. We don't have to analyze our every thought or action to figure out if it might be sin. If you are sinning, you will know if you are willing to listen. There are, however, times in our past where we may have greatly sinned against God and never confessed it or repented. We may have moved on, but that offense toward God remains. Whether it is past or present, be willing to see it and the Lord will be faithful to make it clear.

Once He does, confess your sin and repent. It's what Jesus died for—to forgive you of it all and, in so doing, to heal you.

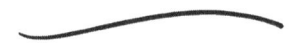

Julia was one of the sweetest ladies I've ever worked with. She came to me with complaints of severe gastrointestinal upset as well as some very bizarre reactions to foods. In our first appointment, she began by sharing her physical symptoms: extreme abdominal pain, gastrointestinal issues, and irregular bowel movements. For the past twelve years she found herself intolerant to most foods and her diet had been whittled down to that of chicken, eggs, steak, and almonds—four foods, that's it. She also reported that she could only eat less than 800 calories a day if she wanted to feel good and function well, which was half the amount she should have been eating.

Her symptoms were severe, and her diet was extreme, but it wasn't anything new to me. I see patients like this all the time. Then came the twist.

Julia reported having some very bizarre emotional reactions to certain foods. The most notable of them was corn. Any trace amount of corn or corn products gave her suicidal thoughts. This reaction was so severe that even generic table salt at restaurants triggered suicidal tendencies because it contained dextrose, a derivative of corn.

Julia grew very serious as she told me this, looking me straight in the eyes as she spoke. "Now I love Jesus… *deeply*. And while I can't wait to be with him in heaven one day, suicide is something I would never, *ever* consider in my right mind."

Her gaze was fixed on me, wanting to be sure I was grasping the weight of what she was saying. She continued. "I love life! But when I consume corn, I become completely consumed with wanting to take my life." Long pause. "I need you to know that this is not normal. This is not me."

It was clear that she genuinely had no desire to harm herself. The suicidal thoughts had been tormenting her for months before she knew that corn was causing them. It was the Lord who finally revealed corn to be the trigger as she was praying one day; and sure enough, when she omitted corn products completely, all the suicidal thoughts stopped.

Not long after the corn reaction was identified and remedied, a new reaction began—extreme fear and paranoia. Through prayer and diligent food tracking, she had determined what foods were triggering these psychological responses and eliminated them from her diet as well. With that, the fear and paranoia went away. Yet, between the gastrointestinal pain being triggered by some foods, and the extreme psychological reactions being caused by others, there was not much left she could eat.

Knowing that I was a Christian, Julia shared with me a bit more about her past. She had been a missionary in 41 different countries throughout her life, some of which had a great deal of spiritual warfare going on. Because of that, she believed something spiritual was likely causing her symptoms. Yet as much as she was aware of that possibility, she had already been through a great deal of spiritual and emotional counseling over the years and received tremendous amounts of prayer, all to no avail. The only thing that physically helped was eliminating foods, and severely restricting her diet.

Julia valued that I wanted to pray and seek the Lord for greater insight into what was going on. However, she had received so much prayer and ministry prior to seeking out my services that now her focus was simply on what practical steps she could take with her diet. This was what she wanted my help with.

I sat and listened, praying for discernment. There was certainly a spiritual aspect to all of this, but I didn't know what it was. I suspected that anything I advised her to do with her diet probably wouldn't help. She requested having a food sensitivity test done, but I was hesitant to add any further restrictions to her already limited food selection. Supplements and nutrient testing might be helpful, but I knew they would only do so much. Nothing in my arsenal of tools seemed ideal. None of my recommendations would likely fix whatever it was that was going on here, so we took it one day at a time.

For months this sweet woman came in to meet with me. Each time, I determined what few dietary recommendations or changes we could make, and then we would pray together. As we prayed, the Holy Spirit would give her a powerful revelation or specific scripture, and both of us would feel greatly encouraged, but still no direct answers came as to why this was all happening. I continued to do my job giving her practical direction with her eating and supplements, but as expected, we didn't see much improvement.

A few weeks later I received a phone call. It was Julia. She was clearly very excited because she was talking so fast that I couldn't make out what she was saying. I listened closely, asking questions, trying to piece it all together, and slowly I began to understand.

Julia woke up that morning with a sudden clarity from the Holy Spirit as to exactly what was making her body so sick. I was beside myself with excitement but could do nothing more than listen—jaw open and mind blown.

Piece by piece, she unfolded a broader story of something that had happened several decades ago. Severe epilepsy had run in her family, and she too had been diagnosed with it when she was young. As she put it, "It was an evil disease that had wrecked the lives of many people I loved, and I was determined that it would go no further."

At that time in her life, Julia didn't know Jesus and believed the only hope she had to cut this disease off from her family was never to have a child to pass it on to. So, in due course, she had herself sterilized.

"Now I know that when I came to Jesus, He forgave me for

everything," she explained, "but this was something that I needed to truly acknowledge and repent for."

Though she couldn't fully explain it, she knew this was the very thing that had robbed her health for so many years. In response, she felt it was important to actually confess and repent before a small group of her close friends.

She called these friends together and confessed to them what she had done so long ago. With them as her witness, she then asked her heavenly Father to forgive her.

Guess what?

All of her symptoms stopped. All of them. She was able to eat anything she wanted without any physical or emotional reaction. God had truly healed her through repentance.

A month later, Julia phoned saying she needed my help again, but she was giggling as she spoke. Apparently, she had spent the entire past month celebrating her restored health by enjoying all the foods she loved with all the people she loved. It had been a month of feasting—savoring her newfound freedom—and she had zero regrets.

Now that the month was over, and she felt she had been able to fully celebrate what God had done, she simply needed me to teach her wisdom. She needed to learn how to eat in a way that nourished her body while also enjoying her life without restrictions.

That I could do.

> **"You kissed my heart with forgiveness in spite of all I've done. You've healed me inside and out from every disease."**
> PSALMS 103:3 (TPT)

The apostle, Paul, speaks of one sin in particular in his letter to the Corinthians, stating it as the reason many had become weak and sick, and some had even died. It wasn't merely unconfessed sin alone, but those who ate the Lord's Supper—or took holy communion—in an unworthy manner.

> "Therefore, whoever eats the bread or drinks the cup of the Lord in an unworthy manner will be guilty of sinning against the body and blood of the Lord. A man ought to examine himself before he eats of the bread and drinks of the cup. For anyone who eats and drinks without recognizing the body of the Lord eats and drinks judgment on himself.
>
> ***That is why many among you are weak and sick***, and a number of you have fallen asleep. But if we judged ourselves, we would not come under judgment. When we are judged by the Lord, ***we are being disciplined so that we will not be condemned with the world.***"
>
> 1 CORINTHIANS 11:27-32 (emphasis mine)

What does it mean to take communion in an unworthy manner? It's referring to the posture of our hearts. Partaking of the Lord's Supper is a very holy privilege. It's a holy covenant—one that we enter into with a holy God who gave His Son so that we could be redeemed. What Jesus did on the cross is no little thing. He was the One God spoke of in the beginning, when sin entered the world—the One who would redeem us back to Him. He was the One the Jews were waiting for for thousands of years. Then Jesus came down from heaven to earth. He loved with an unimaginable love, with extravagant grace and mercy to a world full of people that didn't deserve it. Then, He died for us.

He went down to hell, where He suffered a full and complete separation from the Father so that He could then conquer death once and for all. Three days later, He rose from the dead. He ascended into heaven, and now anyone who believes in Him shall not perish but have eternal life. This is our covenant. We enter into communion acknowledging that His death and resurrection redeemed us.

As such, communion ought never to be taken in a way that we defile it with irreverence. We should not take it with unconfessed sin abiding within us. If we are irreverent or unrepentant, it's like drinking all the judgment and punishment that Jesus carried on the cross back onto ourselves.

Communion is not an antidote for sin. That's what confession and repentance are for and they need to be done first. Communion is holy—not to be invaded with our unconfessed sin, nor with irreverence, apathy, or indifference. It is not an act meant to be taken ritualistically, but one meant to intertwine our hearts as one with His.

It is *the* most priceless and powerful covenant we could ever enter into.

Do not take communion hastily or half-heartedly. Pause. Examine your heart. Confessed and repented-of sin is forgiven sin. Let the sacrifice He made, the price He paid, and the victory He gained be honored by keeping that space sacred. Your health, as well as your spirit, will be blessed for it.

Pray like David prayed:

> "Search me, O God, and know my heart;
> test me and know my anxious thoughts.
> See if there is any offensive way in me,
> and lead me in the way everlasting."
> PSALM 139:23-24

If David's words from Psalm 139 become the daily posture of our hearts, we will find that sin has very little time to exist in our lives before we see it and repent of it. Let's be sure to judge ourselves well, to pay attention to our hearts, our actions, and our thoughts, so as to bring any unholy thing under the blood and covering of Jesus before we fall under the weight of our sin.

If you find that you are facing health challenges that stem from some sort of hidden and unconfessed sin, confess it—whether by yourself or with others bearing witness. Let the amazing grace of Jesus wash over you anew and know that He paid for it all.

Any sickness that is a result of unconfessed sin will depart once it is brought into the light to meet the precious blood of our Savior. A good diet, proper supplementation, and healthy lifestyle can accomplish a lot, but they cannot make us right with God. They cannot give our bodies the life that comes from His blessing.

Now, a word of caution. Don't go looking for something that isn't there. If God doesn't highlight something specifically, don't continue to introspectively over-analyze your thoughts and your life to find every hint of potential sin that might need to be dealt with. When you do this, you take your eyes off Jesus and put them on yourself. If God wants to show you something, just pay attention. You will see it. Look at Him and, in time, He will show you if it's there. If He does not impress your heart with anything, move on.

Keep it simple. Live your life in love with Him. Posture your heart like David did, and allow Him to lead you as He will.

chapter 19

afflictions

To quote Heidi Baker once more, "Satan is trying to destroy your destiny, God's temple. If he can't use sin, he will use sickness or exhaustion. So we have to fight" (*Reckless Devotion*). The enemy will do anything He can to try and hinder us, distract us, and discourage us from the Lord and His Kingdom.

Satan loves to go after our health, all the while trying to convince us it is a physical issue that we are responsible to fix. For our purposes, we will call this a spiritual affliction—a health issue caused solely by the enemy. It can be anything from pain to nagging symptoms or disease, but the only way to overcome it is through Jesus. Medicine, diet, supplements, and other therapies may help or provide some temporary relief; but, if it's an affliction from the enemy, the only way to ultimately heal is through the blood of Jesus forcing that affliction to leave.

First understand that you have a destiny. You have been set apart by God for a divine purpose. You have a choice to pursue that destiny and, with that pursuit, you will experience opposition—both in the world and in the spirit realm. The greatest fear the enemy has is that you will reach the full potential for which God created you. Why should we be surprised when our physical bodies are an object of his attempts to hinder us?

Evil isn't really that profound. The enemy can be sneaky and subtle at times, but his ways are not profound. His tactics are always to steal, kill and destroy, and he looks for any opportunity possible to do just that. While we don't want to focus too much on the enemy and what evil is trying to do, make no mistake: we want to be aware of it so that we don't fall prey to it. With these attacks on our health, it may feel like he is winning at times, but there will always be victory in Christ if we fight for it.

Take a look at the words Jesus spoke to his disciples after He first sent them out to minister to people.

> "The seventy-two returned with joy and said, 'Lord, even the demons submit to us in your name.'
>
> He replied, 'I saw Satan fall like lightning from heaven. I have given you authority to trample on snakes and scorpions and to overcome all the power of the enemy; nothing will harm you. However, do not rejoice that the spirits submit to you, but rejoice that your names are written in heaven.'"
>
> LUKE 10:17-20

We don't have to be afraid of the enemy or his tactics. If we are in Christ Jesus, we have authority over anything and everything Satan does; we have power over Satan himself. He would like us to think we don't. When the health battle gets long and isn't won in a victorious moment, we can become easily convinced that we are at his mercy. Remember Who it is that lives within us.

This authority to trample the enemy has to be exercised. It's not passive, and it doesn't happen by accident. If we discern that what we are experiencing is an attack, we must focus and declare what is true—which is often the very opposite of what seems to be true in the moment. In doing so, we will disarm everything meant to harm us.

I've experienced a handful of these types of afflictions over the last several years, and I've seen a couple of patients walk through them as well. There are two different reasons for them that I've come to understand: either it is purely an attack, or it is the result of some agreement we have made with the enemy.

The first, an attack from the enemy, occurs through nothing of our own doing. Evil is launching an assault against us in an attempt to break us—to steal our hope, disconnect us from Jesus, rob our freedom, and ultimately keep us from our destiny.

There is nothing we have done that causes these attacks to happen. We didn't do anything that gave opportunity to the enemy; it wasn't our fault. But if the Lord allowed it, it's because He knows it will only serve to test and prove our faith, to strengthen us and grow us all the more. These moments, these trials, will become memorial stone moments where, like the disciples, we come back to Jesus in awe of the authority we have been given to overcome.

What matters is not why the attack happened, but how we respond to it. The first step is to discern that what you are facing is, in fact, an attack. It doesn't mean that the physical issue you are up against isn't real in your physical body, but it means it isn't your responsibility to fix it. I've seen this come in the form of something as simple as joint pain or an upset stomach, or as severe as a life-altering disease.

Let me be clear. Not fixing yourself doesn't necessarily mean you don't do something to care for your physical body—medically or naturally or nutritionally. It isn't a sin to take actionable steps for relief, though there may be times when Jesus asks you not to. We can seek to change our diet, our lifestyle, or get help in any number of ways, but we know that none of it will ultimately heal us of these afflictions for good. It can, however, help sustain us until the spiritual victory comes and that affliction finally leaves.

These are not battles of flesh and blood, but ones that are "against the powers of this dark world and against the spiritual forces of evil in the heavenly realms" (Ephesians 6:12). As such, whether or not you tend to your physical health with any physical support isn't what matters or where the actual victory lies. Victory here will only be won by the blood of Jesus, and by us exercising our authority in Him.

What does it look like to exercise our authority? We use our words, our prayers, our thoughts, and our actions to declare truth over our bodies and over the situation. Ask the Lord for wisdom to know how to pray and what to speak.

Everything the enemy does is an attempt to contradict truth. If he can put tiny cracks in the foundations of our beliefs, little by little he knows we will start to lose our footing. It is imperative that we anchor ourselves to Jesus in truth because everything the enemy does tempts us to believe a lie. So we must think, pray, and speak things that are true—words that are full of life, even if everything we are experiencing feels contrary to it. This requires great faith in the unseen promises of God, and it is profoundly powerful. Our words and our thoughts have more authority to impact change than we can possibly understand—in the world, in our bodies, in our minds, and in the spirit realm. This is the authority that Jesus spoke of.

When we are anchored in truth and focused on Jesus, we can then see all the pits the enemy tries to lure us into much more clearly. It may be the pit of discouragement, of hopelessness, of self-pity, of striving, of accepting the lie that this is just how it is. The pit of accepting a diagnosis that isn't really ours to carry, or of fear. Or, to quote the Princess Bride, "the pit of despair." Lots of pits, zero help.

When we can see a pit, we can avert our focus to avoid falling into it. Think about it like riding a bike. If you see a pothole, don't look at it or you will inevitably hit it. Choose instead to look where you want to go, and your bike will follow. Likewise, don't narrow in on the health issue. Don't become consumed with what the enemy is doing. Look to Jesus and ask Him what He is doing. Keep believing His promises, and consider speaking them out loud over your body, over your destiny, over anything you feel compelled to.

Because many of these pits have to do with our thoughts, it's vitally important that we choose carefully what we believe. I've fallen, and at times willingly climbed, into those pits more than I care to admit because I didn't guard my thoughts. Usually I didn't see the pit until I was in it. Sometimes the pit felt more comforting—until it didn't.

Eventually, after enough pits, I began to see how destructive and miserable they were. Not only did they suck the life out of me, but they also took a lot more time and effort to climb out of than if I had never gone down in the first place. I had to open my eyes and learn to see the choices I was making in my thoughts based on what I was experiencing with my body. When I finally understood the gravity of them, I was strengthened to choose different thoughts, to speak better things, to hold on to truth rather than doubt. Soon enough, victory, hope, and peace became my normal companions.

If you are facing a health issue that you sense is a spiritual attack, choose today how you will respond in faith. Then choose again tomorrow, and the next day, and the next, until that cursed thing leaves. And trust me, with Jesus, it will. But it doesn't always happen right away.

Sometimes we have to contend for victory. That affliction may leave the instant you speak the name of Jesus over it, or it might not. Don't be discouraged if it's more of a journey than you thought. Anchor yourself to Jesus, and then stand firm in His truth. Standing firm, in my opinion, is one of the most challenging acts of faith because it goes against everything visible to trust God for all that is not yet seen. This is where faith truly gets activated—"when we are hard pressed on every side, but not crushed; perplexed, but not in despair; persecuted, but not abandoned; struck down, but not destroyed" (2 Corinthians 4:8-9).

> **"Therefore put on the full armor of God, so that when the day of evil comes, you may be able to stand your ground, and *after you have done everything, to stand*. Stand firm then..."**
> EPHESIANS 6:13-14 (emphasis mine)

It seems so simple—standing firm—especially in a health culture that has become so complex and demanding about what you must do to be healed. It may even seem irresponsible, which is perhaps the greatest struggle many people have in getting victory. Standing firm is a powerful testimony to the enemy that you know Who lives inside of you. It's not passive; it is a powerful choice.

In the end—once victory has come, the affliction has left, and we are physically healed—it will have drawn the roots of our faith deeper. Deeper than they ever could have gone on their own. The only reason the Lord would allow the enemy to attack us in these instances is because He knows we are capable of overcoming and, in the overcoming, we will be more propelled toward becoming fully who God created us to be than if we had never been afflicted in the first place. What was meant to harm us, God will turn for our good. The enemy's ways may not be profound, but the ways of the Lord are wonderfully profound.

If you think back to the story of Job, he had to endure these evil afflictions for a time, but only for a time (Read Job 1-2 for more background to his story). The Lord allowed it to test him, to produce greater endurance and perseverance in him, and then victory came—suddenly and powerfully. In the end, more was restored to Job than was lost. This is our promise too. He is faithful.

Several years ago, I sat in my favorite tea shop, across the table from a dear friend. Despite how much I was enjoying our time together, I was constantly fidgeting, unable to get comfortable. My back throbbed and my hips were aching. It had been a month of this awful pain coming and going, sometimes in my neck, sometimes in my hips, or in other parts of my back. I never thought much about it until it began affecting my ability to sit for even short periods of time. Standing was just as painful after a few minutes, so I soon became uncomfortable no matter what I did.

I went to a wonderful chiropractor who discovered my muscles were incredibly tense and spasming at times. The tension was pulling on my bones, causing my hips and spine to be constantly pulled out of alignment. He assigned me different stretches and coached me through proper sitting to avoid back or neck strain. I was told to stop all weight-bearing workouts and focus only on aerobic exercise.

For months I went in for regular adjustments, got some massages, practiced perfect posture, and minimized my workouts to simply walking. It all seemed to help. My muscles did calm down some—but the pain never fully went away.

Eventually, being the dietitian that I am, I cut out sugar. Out of curiosity, I wanted to see if it was related, and much to my surprise all the tension and pain seemed to go away within a few days. Hallelujah!

This seemed to be the answer, and yet deep down I wrestled with it. I wasn't eating irresponsibly, nor was I eating much sugar to begin with. I felt no conviction from the Holy Spirit to avoid sugar altogether, nor did I feel peaceful or content about making the change. Yet if I ate sugar, the tension would return, and the pain would increase. Some days it was my neck, some days it was my back, some days it was my hip—the pain never seemed to settle in one place, but it never failed to present itself like a nagging, unwelcome companion.

One night I laid awake in bed as the pain began to throb. Not wanting to wake Nathan, I went downstairs and stretched out on the couch.

"God, what is this?" I whispered in desperation.

Immediately I heard Him answer. "It's a messenger of Satan sent to afflict and torment you."

Whaaaat? My eyes went wide. This was the last thing I ever expected to hear from the Lord, probably because I had never experienced something like it before.

Hearing this, I boldly told that messenger to leave, knowing full well that I had authority to do so in the name of Jesus. I spoke the blood of Jesus over me with every ounce of faith I had, and yet the pain remained.

It would seem discouraging, not seeing the affliction leave at the authority of my prayers—and perhaps it was on some level—but oddly I still felt liberated. If this was an affliction from the enemy and I was asking Jesus for help, then He would be faithful. It was no longer my problem to figure out, but Jesus' problem to answer.

The pain continued to come and go over the next few weeks, affecting different areas at different times. Each chiropractor visit would continually verify that my physical body was out of alignment, despite the fact that now I knew it was a spiritual cause. I often wondered if I had heard the Lord wrong, or just thought it up on my own. It's so easy to doubt the Lord's voice in the waiting. Some of the greatest tests of my faith have been in times of waiting.

The physical struggles continued. Sometimes it was incredibly painful and all consuming. Other times it was tolerable and I could ignore it. I did my best to support myself with physical care—sitting and standing properly, stretching, and eating well. However, I gave up on avoiding all sugar because I now knew it was a lie that sugar was the source of the pain.

Some time later, I was at a women's retreat in the mountains. One night, as the speaker finished his session, he said, "There are about ten people in this room who have a pain that migrates between your neck, back, and hips."

I perked right up, eyes wide. This was for me. After months and months of pain, I could feel hope swelling within me that something was finally about to change.

"That pain is an afflicting spirit, and it is afflicting you because you are called to be intercessors."

My jaw dropped.

So I didn't hear the Lord wrong. I thought. *It is an afflicting spirit.*

The speaker proceeded to have anyone stand who felt that the prophetic revelation was for them, and I was the first one on my feet. He prayed over us, though I can't really remember what He prayed, and then asked us to agree with our calling as intercessors. I did, though I had never thought of myself as such before. We all said amen, and that was that.

Two mornings later, when I woke up, I twisted my body to do my usual morning stretch. As I did, every vertebra in my back popped from bottom to top like a zipper going up my spine. With it, every ounce of pain left.

A few days later, I went in for my weekly chiropractor visit. He did his usual assessment, and I waited for his typical banter about what was out of line and how badly. Everything felt amazing, but I didn't know what to expect him to find.

"What have you been doing?" he asked with great surprise. "Your hips and neck are perfectly in line!" He was shocked and incredibly curious as to what had changed.

Never in my life has a chiropractor told me my hips are in line. In high school, my chiropractor discovered that I had one leg slightly longer than the other, which caused my hips to be misaligned and problematic. When I heard my chiropractor now say that my hips were actually in line, as well as my back and neck, all I could do was laugh in amazement.

All that pain was never mine to own. It was not a result of me doing anything wrong or needing to do anything differently. I simply needed God to set me free in His way and in His time. All the physical things I did to find relief—the chiropractic care, reduced sugar intake, stretching, and good posture—were not wrong or a waste of my time. In fact, these are practices that I have continued to some degree over the years. But they were not the crux of the issue; it was an afflicting spirit.

What the enemy never counted on—through his attack on my physical body in an attempt to undermine my calling as an intercessor—was that God would illuminate my calling even more clearly. All that the pain tried to hinder and destroy was only magnified all the more in the end.

Affliction, laid before Jesus, will always accomplish far greater things than it tries to hinder. That, my friends, is the beautifully redemptive nature of Jesus.

The second type of spiritual affliction happens when we come into an agreement with Satan. It may be through lies we choose to believe, or permissions we give him—whether or not we realize it. Or it may be through occultic practices, past or present.

Rather than the enemy going after our health in an effort to find a way into our heart, this second type of affliction starts with an open door in our hearts that the enemy then uses to afflict our health, which then further cripples our hearts. At some point, we gave him permission to afflict us by coming into agreement with him—usually through taking hold of a lie. He is, after all, the father of lies. The more we grow in discernment—the more we learn to take our thoughts captive and think on things that are good and true—the less the enemy will find a way in.

God often speaks to me through dreams. There was one year in particular in which He was teaching me the vital importance of my beliefs and agreements. It was a year where I felt the constant attack of the enemy on every side—in my health, mindset, and relationships. Even my time with Jesus felt empty and I found it painfully difficult to connect with Him. I became angry with God because it felt like He was no longer protecting me. In my mind, it was His fault I was struggling.

Then came the dream:

I was with my husband, Jesus. I had my back to Him, unable to see Him as He watched and listened to me talk to someone else.

"I don't know how to be intimate with Him," I told the other person that I was facing. "I honestly don't even think I like it. It's uncomfortable, and I think I need to go elsewhere for intimacy."

I spoke while Jesus listened behind me, though I didn't know He was there. He was bent over, elbows on his knees, head sunken, as though his heart was breaking. The sorrow in His face was immeasurable, as was the depth of love He had for me; but at that time, I didn't know how to receive His love.

Jesus did not speak or interject. He would never force me, His beloved, to be intimate with Him, but He desperately wanted me to choose Him. In the dream, I believed it was His fault that I couldn't connect with Him, but clearly it was my choice.

Then, still oblivious to Jesus behind me, I stood up and walked to a nearby door. I knocked on the door and, much to my surprise, a prostitute answered. I was a little shocked, but even still, I didn't close the door. Rather I stood there, considering all she had to offer me. Then I woke up.

When my eyes opened, I remembered the dream and conviction instantly pierced my heart. All I could do was repent over and over and over.

"Forgive me Jesus. I'm so sorry."

It was the first time I realized what was happening. I had forsaken my intimacy with Jesus and had opened the door to the enemy—the prostitute—with my thoughts. Two things struck me—how on earth I could think a prostitute would give me anything worth wanting but, even more so, how deeply my Jesus loved me.

I had believed these lies that it was His fault I couldn't connect with Him. But, in reality, I was choosing to believe lies for a false sense of comfort instead of being with Him. Practically what that looked like was me allowing my circumstances to provoke my thoughts towards frustration, bitterness, anger, entitlement, and so on. It felt more comforting to get upset and bothered than to find a way to be grateful. Out of the darkness of my heart, my mouth then spoke. I complained, I grumbled, I blamed. I wasn't careful with my words, or how I was responding to these trials, and it had given the enemy an open door into my life. As a result, I was constantly dealing with my old health issues again.

The dream was shocking, but I needed to see it to understand the weight of what I was choosing to think, to believe, and to speak. You see, it's not just about opening the door to the enemy or what health affliction may come. It's about our connection to Jesus. Every lie we believe or agreement we make with the enemy steals our intimacy with the One we love—the One who loves us more deeply than we can ever fathom.

If you find yourself dealing with a health issue that seems to be a spiritual affliction, ask the Lord to show you if there is any way you have been partnering with the enemy or His lies. What the enemy doesn't realize is that this type of spiritual affliction is also a tool to grow us in truth. The more we can see these afflictions when they come, the quicker we will be to repent and then choose to dwell on what is good and pure. This is how we renew our mind in Christ.

Two things had to happen after that dream. I had to close the door to the lies, and I had to turn back to Jesus. This is true of any time we have unknowingly partnered with the enemy—from a small lie to the occult. Repentance and returning are our restoration.

Tori came to me with a long list of symptoms: severe stomach pain, brain fog, blurry vision, sporadic vomiting, body aches, irritable bowel symptoms, and constant feelings of coldness. She had been through a lot of medical issues in the previous fifteen years and had been diagnosed with two autoimmune diseases.

Her symptoms were not uncommon, and for the most part, they could be physically explained. What was most astounding, however, was her reaction to water. Drinking any amount of water would cause her to vomit it back up, so she stopped drinking it altogether. Water, the very liquid that is a source of life for our bodies and constitutes 60% of our body mass, was something she couldn't consume. Instead, she drank milk—a lot of milk.

Alarm bells were going off in my spirit, and I knew this was not just about physical issues. Discernment was telling me that something spiritual was at work here against her, but I was completely at a loss for what to do.

Not only is water necessary for our physical body to function but, all throughout scripture, water is also depicted as a source of life. The opposite is true as well. In Matthew 12:43, we read that evil spirits live in a waterless realm where there is no rest. Here Tori was, completely incapable of drinking water. Was it related? Was there something evil afflicting her?

I sat across the desk from Tori, listening to her share while also praying for wisdom. This was way beyond what I had ever come across. If I could turn off my spiritual discernment and just focus on the physical issues at hand, there was a lot that I could reason to do. The water reaction, however, confounded all my natural wisdom. It was baffling unless I looked at it through a spiritual lens. Then, perhaps, it made some sense. I simply couldn't ignore my gnawing sense that this was something that needed spiritual attention.

The Holy Spirit then whispered:

> **"The afflicted and needy are seeking water, but there is none, and their tongues are parched with thirst; I, the Lord, will answer them Myself, as the God of Israel I will not forsake them."**
>
> ISAIAH 41:17 (NASB)

I didn't have much time to ponder this, but I instinctively knew the Lord was telling me there was, in fact, something more than dietary issues at play. This was spiritual, at least some part of it, and He was about to answer.

I'm not really sure how it all happened, but I ended up sharing the gospel with her. I talked to her about the things of God and the things of Satan, describing a spiritual war that we often can't see but that we can very much feel—one that can sometimes affect our physical health. Things were coming out of my mouth that I was quite shocked by—not because they were wrong, but because I was a professional. How was I sitting here talking to a patient, who I knew was not a Christian, about spiritual warfare?

Nonetheless, I had to say something. Surprisingly, everything I said struck a deep chord in her. She listened attentively, and then was silent. It may have been the longest moment of silence I've ever experienced. How is it that I can be so sure I needed to say something, and yet so terrified that I was saying the wrong thing?

Finally, Tori spoke. She began telling me about a relationship from fifteen years ago with a man that had been a devout Satan worshipper. It was a serious relationship, but she was not a part of the occult like he was.

At this point, my eyes must have been the size of walnuts. I said nothing and let her continue to talk.

"He got further and further into the occult," She said, "and I hated it. So one day, I finally had enough and told Satan, 'Leave him alone! You deal with me now.'"

I could see the wheels turning in her mind as she shared and processed all of this. "You know," she said, "it was about that time that all these health issues started."

I was stunned. Completely in shock. No words came out of my mouth but my spirit within me was still praying ferociously.

Tori continued thinking, "It feels like I am at a fork in the road and I have to choose which direction I want to go."

She processed out loud about the idea of salvation and Jesus, amazed that no one had ever told her about these things before. Those several minutes felt like an eternity as I sat and listened, praying and praying for her to choose Jesus.

Suddenly she spoke.

"Okay, let's do it! What do we do? Do we get down on our knees and pray?"

I think my heart completely skipped a beat at that moment. *Is this really happening?* I thought. She was so childlike, so eager to pray. I couldn't help but chuckle at how precious it was.

"Sure, we can pray however you want to," I responded.

Before I could blink, she pushed the chairs out of the way and dropped to her knees. I came around the desk and knelt down next to her. Once we were both face to face on our knees, she looked into my eyes and said with a bit of sadness, "My eyes used to have light in them like your eyes do. I want that again."

I smiled. "You will soon."

I led her in words to pray. She repeated them, but said everything in her own words, through tears, and with such gratitude and brokenness. Tears welled up in my eyes each time Tori spoke. With every step of that prayer her heart seemed to be more and more overwhelmed by God's love. By the time we said amen, she just sat there on her knees, weeping, saying, "Thank you Jesus. Thank you, Jesus. Thank you, Jesus," over and over and over. It was a holy moment like I had never experienced before.

When her eyes finally opened, soaked through with tears of gratitude, there was light in them. There was so much brightness and life in her eyes and her face that I was undone.

Only Jesus. I am so thankful that my spirit wouldn't let me just focus on Tori's physical needs when her spirit needed to be healed and set free first.

I kept in touch with Tori for a few months after that. She got plugged into a wonderful church and started taking classes to learn more about life with Jesus. I fully expected all of her health issues to resolve as a result. They did improve tremendously, but they did not fully resolve. Certain foods still bothered her, which was quite disappointing for me at the time.

I wish I knew back then what I know now. I thought that if Tori's health issues were a result of spiritual issues, then any physical support for healing was unnecessary. While this can be true for some, there are times when both are important and necessary. The afflicting hand of the enemy needs to be removed first, but the body might still need physical support and time to recover from the effects of that affliction. Tori had faced this affliction for fifteen years, and it was going to take some time for her body to get back to normal. Now, however, healing was possible.

Our health journeys may have layers to them. Jesus is faithful to take us through them one step at a time, leaving nothing out, until one day we look back and realize how far we have come. Spiritual afflictions may be the sole cause of a health issue or one huge piece of it. Either way, we can find comfort in remembering that Jesus knows what we need when we need it. Spiritual afflictions may be a part of our story, but it's the victory over those afflictions that we will remember and be forever marked by.

chapter 20

emotions

In ancient Greek culture, the bowels, or intestines, were described as the seat of emotions. In ancient Jewish culture, the Hebrew word for anguish and bowels can be used interchangeably. Today, what the Greeks and Jews surmised by observation, we now validate with science. The intensity of emotion changes how the body functions completely, and thus our emotions can significantly impact our health.

We are meant to feel. It means our hearts are very much alive, even if what we are feeling is hard or heavy. Some emotions will strengthen our bodies and promote rest and healing—things like joy, peace, hope, and gratitude. This is where we want to posture our hearts and strive to be.

The reality, however, is that life isn't always easy and, though we can contend for peace, hope, joy, and gratitude, we may have to walk through valleys to get there. We will face challenging, unpleasant emotions as well—emotions such as grief, trauma, pain, heartache, anxiety, depression, anger, fear, and worry. No one longs to feel these things, but they are inevitable. In a world where the enemy roams, where sin and brokenness exist, where we age and death happens, these emotions are real.

Both sets of emotions can impact our health, but how do we navigate them so they don't navigate us? Let's start with understanding what physically happens as a response to those emotions.

Each of us is equipped with an autonomic nervous system that has two parts: the sympathetic and parasympathetic nervous systems. The sympathetic nervous system activates our bodies towards a "fight or flight" response. It slows digestion and tissue repair and redirects the body's energy toward other functions, thus preparing for an emergency—think *adrenaline*. Heart rate increases, blood vessels constrict, blood pressure increases, and breathing quickens as various hormones are released. As this happens, daily restorative functions—like digestion, healing, and tissue repair—get mildly or massively hindered.

The "fight or flight" response is a very necessary part of a healthy body. When God created us, he knew we would face things that require our body to supercharge itself for action or help get us through challenging moments or circumstances. It's not a bad thing. But too much time in "fight or flight" puts more and more stress on the body as it tries to cope with whatever emotional or physical stress we are experiencing.

On the other hand, the parasympathetic nervous system shifts the functional systems of the body towards a more relaxed "rest and digest" response. Stress on the body is reduced, digestive functions are enhanced, and restorative functions that promote healing are optimized.

We are always functioning between the two sides of the autonomic nervous system, sometimes more to one side than the other. They are both a necessary part of a healthy body, but too much time in "fight or flight" will start to drain and break down the body physically. New health issues can arise—or existing ones can worsen—as a result.

Emotions and physical stimuli trigger how your autonomic nervous system will respond. If you feel stress, grief, fear, anxiety, worry, heartsickness, or any difficult emotional response, your body will swing more towards the "fight or flight" side. You will also find yourself in "fight or flight" if you are constantly operating on adrenaline and working in overdrive—even if you're doing things you love. If you experience peace, hope, joy, contentment, or rest, your body adjusts towards the "rest and digest" side where it can restore, heal, and thrive.

Just because it is more ideal to be in the calming and restorative side of the autonomic nervous system doesn't mean it's unhealthy to swing to the stress and adrenaline side at times. There is a time for each response and the emotions that come with them. There is a season for everything. These two parts of the autonomic nervous system are meant to exist in a healthy tension.

Too much of the heightened joy and adrenaline rush of life can push us out of balance as well. As such, we have to come back to knowing our season. We have to come back to wisdom, discerning what our bodies need.

Hard emotions and physical stress do not always cause health issues, but they can. Your body can handle a lot before it starts to break down and show physical signs of wear. Whether or not your physical health is being affected by too much emotional stress, it's still good to learn how to navigate it. Health issues will give us all the more motivation to do so.

I've found myself more and more grateful for the times when my body is impacted by my emotions. It's a wakeup call. In those times, I'm probably leaning more on my own strength than the One who is my strength, my own comforts than the One who is my comfort.

If there is a storm I'm feeling and I'm being rocked, clearly I've yet to find my peace in the midst of the storm—Jesus. He is always there, in the midst of the emotional turbulence of life, just waiting for us to lean on Him rather than ourselves. When we do, those hard emotions and all that responsibility we carry are suddenly pierced with the good emotions. Fear gets pierced with peace, sorrow gives way to joy, stillness and rest are found in the midst of the storm. It doesn't make sense to our minds, but that's what's so magnificent about a God whose ways are so much greater than our own. It doesn't make sense, but that doesn't make it any less real.

We can experience a variety of unpleasant emotions for an infinite number of reasons. Some causes we have control over and need to deal with. Other times, the root of our emotions is something we can't change, and the only way past our emotions is to walk through them.

First, let's start with what we have control over. Our emotions can be a passive thing if we let them, where our feelings directly relate to our circumstances. It's like being tossed by every wind and wave that comes our way. Or, we can recognize what we're feeling, identify why we're feeling it, and then get to the root of the truth needed to help us overcome it.

Work, politics, relationships, circumstances—life is prone to storms. But perhaps we exacerbate the storms by how we respond to them. The disciples knew this well.

> "That day when evening came, he said to his disciples, 'Let us go over to the other side.' Leaving the crowd behind, they took him along, just as he was, in the boat. There were also other boats with him. A furious squall came up, and the waves broke over the boat, so that it was nearly swamped. Jesus was in the stern, sleeping on a cushion. The disciples woke him and said, 'Teacher, don't you care if we drown?'
>
> He got up, rebuked the wind and said to the waves, 'Quiet! Be still!' Then the wind died down and it was completely calm. He said to his disciples, 'Why are you so afraid? Do you still have no faith?'"
>
> MARK 4:35-40

Those last words always send a chill up my spine in the best way possible. Do we need Jesus to come in and ask us, "What are you so afraid of? Do you still have no faith?"

Many of those unpleasant emotions can stem from fear. Fear of *what* is the question. Negative emotions are not things we can merely recognize and then turn off like a light switch. They have to be recognized and then replaced with something better—something bigger. They have to be replaced with a truth more powerful than our feelings or circumstances: a truth that can anchor us, guide us, and lead us. A truth we can stand on.

It's in those times that we need to hear from the Lord. We need Him to speak to us, to encourage our hearts, and to remind us of what is true. Filling our minds with the voice of God breathes life back into our hearts. For every unpleasant emotion, there is truth waiting to be found, or rediscovered, to help us overcome it. God wants to speak into our storms, but we have to make the active choice to seek Him and listen.

Once He speaks, we need to align our thoughts, our words, and our actions with that truth. If we continue speaking about the things that stress us out, reacting to the storms in our flesh, then our emotions will follow. Our bodies and health will follow.

Hard as it may be, we have to speak the things that Jesus is speaking and do the things that line up with His words. Speak what is good, hopeful, true, and life giving. Find tangible ways to help you stay in that heavenly mindset as you go about your life.

Over the years, I've worked with a handful of patients that I just could not help, no matter how compliant they were. These patients lived in a constant state of anxiety and worry, and the stress was taking a massive toll on their health. Some of their emotions were justified, as they had lived through a lot of trauma that continued to inform their thoughts and perspectives. Others, however, chose to consider these emotions as a part of who they were, with no desire to change.

"I'm just a worrier." "I am an anxious person; I've just always been that way." This mindset accepted these negative emotions as a part of their identity. There was no hope for overcoming the emotions; they only wanted to know how I could help them fix their bodies with food.

These were some of my more challenging patients because it always felt like we were running in place: no ground gained, fighting hard to get nowhere.

As a dietitian, my reach only goes so far. If the negative emotions and mindsets become an acceptable way of life, then there is only so much we can do to help the body manage that type of stress load. The truth is, no one was created to be an "anxious person." Anxiety is a byproduct of something, as are fear and worry, bitterness, anger, and the like. We can't settle for these as being a part of our character or an acceptable part of our lives. Remember, as believers of Jesus Christ, the standard set for us is love, joy, peace, patience, and hope. We must choose to move forward, believe God for more, and then fight for it. He may give us a physical answer—nutrient deficiencies, poor diet, hormones, etc—but, even in those answers, we have to anchor into truth.

Any negative emotion can push our body towards that "fight or flight" way of functioning. We have a choice: are we going to own the negative emotions or are we going to choose to fight for something better? To seek wisdom to overcome? Once the choice has been made, even if it takes time, treating the physical body will often become much more effective as the body is able to calm down and heal.

We are called to live from a heavenly perspective and, from that place with Jesus, the world and its flaws will seem much more benign than we once thought. Jesus demonstrated His authority over the wind and the waves in the boat that day. That same authority lives within us. Our emotions can toss us to and fro like the waves of the sea if we let them. Maybe we need to learn how to respond like Jesus did. Rise up, speak to the waves and the wind and the sea. "Quiet! Be still!" Because Jesus is always bigger than the storm.

Not every unpleasant emotion is one we can overcome with words and prayer alone. Some challenging emotions, such as grief, heartache, trauma, and sorrow, often have to be felt to be able to move past them. There's no way around; only through.

We can choose to ignore the emotions and pretend they aren't there, swallowing them and allowing them to take up residence deep within the crevices of our souls. There they will eat away at our spirits and our bodies, holding us captive until we face them. We can also go to the other extreme and choose to embrace the negative emotions so much that we set up camp in the pit with them. This also holds us captive, unable to heal and move forward.

No matter how much it hurts or how overwhelming it might be, we must choose to face the pain by looking to Jesus, moving gradually through it, and allowing Him to comfort and strengthen us every step of the way.

In these seasons, our physical bodies will often feel the impact of our emotions. Grief, anguish, sorrow, and the like can, at times, be more than our human bodies can handle. Think about Jesus in the garden praying, anticipating his upcoming torturous death. He was in such emotional agony that he sweat blood—a perfect—and somewhat difficult—example of how greatly our emotions can impact our physical bodies.

> **"An angel from heaven appeared to him and strengthened him. And being *in anguish*, he prayed more earnestly, and his sweat was like drops of blood falling to the ground."**
> LUKE 22:43-44 (emphasis mine)

God in heaven sent his angel to strengthen Jesus before the most painful hours of his life. Even with the strength from this angelic visitation, his soul was still in anguish. Jesus knew what awaited him—the horrific pain he would endure, the weight of our sin he would carry, the sorrow of death.

Much as He knew these things, He also knew the endgame. He knew that He would rise up from the grave, death would be defeated, and salvation would be ours. Knowing that it would all turn out for good didn't eliminate the load Jesus carried, but I imagine it did lighten it. It didn't take away the anguish but, in the midst of it, hope hovered.

Sometimes we think that, because we have the hope of Jesus and trust in Him, we shouldn't feel the hard feelings too much. That's simply not true. Jesus knew He would conquer death yet still felt every ounce of emotion in anticipation of it.

Odds are, you and I have not suffered to the point of sweating blood, but we have faced impossibly hard things. We have all felt the pangs of our emotions in challenging times, big or small, and may have also felt the physical toll they've taken.

First, I can't say it enough—have lots of grace for yourself. Ask the Lord to help you through the valley, to give you supernatural hope, peace, and joy, even in the midst of the pain, anguish, or grief. Determine how you can best care for yourself in a way that is realistic and life-giving in those seasons. You may or may not have the capacity for a lot of diet changes and strict self-care, so find what you do have the capacity for. It's true that the body could use some extra care and support in stressful times, but it may not be in the ways you immediately think. Even the best diet and perfect workout regimen isn't beneficial if it only adds stress to an already stressed body and soul. Be discerning about what you take on and what you let go of. You may just need comfort through food. You may need the freedom to simply eat what's available. You may need to rest more and do less. Remember that wisdom changes with the seasons.

Only the Lord knows what you need, and you are the one He will tell; you are the one He will lead. He's not going to reveal these things to anyone but you, even if He uses other people to speak, teach, or give input and ideas that help you find the wisdom you need. You are the one to test and discern what is good and right for you in those times.

I often work with patients who have been through seasons of trauma, pain, grief, or emotional stress that was beyond their control. Some are still in those seasons and, for them, we take things slow and with a lot of grace, addressing both the physical needs of the body as well as the emotional wellbeing of the heart.

Others have already made it through the hard emotions and have come out the other side, yet the body still needs to heal. While the body can restore and heal on its own after emotional stress is gone, there are times when the trauma of it all may have depleted the body beyond its capacity to fully heal on its own. It might need a little help. In these cases, we focus on what still isn't working properly, why, and what nutrition and lifestyle adjustments are needed to support this final phase of healing.

The journey through pain and intense emotions will vary in its duration. Trying to force ourselves to heal and move forward too quickly can be just as detrimental as not healing at all. The Lord knows the way through; we just have to follow one little or big step at a time.

Let go of expectations and have a lot of grace for yourself. It's okay to not feel okay if you know you are headed in the right direction. Just choose to move forward.

In John 11, when Martha's brother, Lazarus, died, she ran to meet Jesus where she fell at his feet and wept.

> "...'Lord, if you had been here, my brother would not have died.'
>
> **When Jesus saw her weeping, and the Jews who had come along with her also weeping, he was deeply moved in spirit and troubled. 'Where have you laid him?' he asked.**
>
> 'Come and see, Lord,' they replied. Jesus wept."
>
> JOHN 11:32-35

Jesus wept. It's a verse many of us know well, but here's what's profound: Jesus knew He was going to resurrect Lazarus. He already knew the endgame here, just like He did when He was in the garden, praying in anguish. He didn't tell Martha, "Hey, it's okay! I'm going to raise him back to life." Nor did He say, "Woman, where is your faith?" Instead, He wept.

The grief and loss and pain that Martha and all the people were feeling was so precious and valuable to Jesus that He wept too. Jesus is always with us in our pain if we are willing to let Him in. Martha ran to Him with hers, and He treasured it. That's our choice too—to turn to Him in our pain, frustration, anger, and hurt—and then let Him breathe the hope back in.

The assurance we have is that for every painful emotion, every challenging time, the Lord is with us in the middle of it. He will get us through to the other side. Because of that valley, we know the beauty of mountaintops all the more.

All the pleasant emotions that give life and healing to our physical bodies are often found by walking through the hard ones. You can't live without them both.

Emotions are powerful. What we feel is important. If you sense that you are experiencing a health issue that is the result of emotion or stress, ask yourself: is this something I need to deal with and overcome? Or is this something I need to walk through?

Fall into the arms of Jesus. He is with you. Let Him into your struggle so He can minister to you. He knows what we're going through more than anyone else ever could.

> **"I have told you these things, so that in me you may have peace. In this world you will have trouble. But take heart! I have overcome the world."**
>
> JOHN 16:33

chapter 21

prophetic insight

> "Carry each other's burdens, and in this way you will fulfill the law of Christ."
>
> GALATIANS 6:2

We may, at times, experience sickness, pain, or other health challenges in order to help someone else. It's not something that is "ours;" we're sharing another person's struggles. This is supernatural.

In these instances, we may be feeling, in part or in whole, what *someone else* is experiencing. That's not to say that what's physically happening in our bodies isn't real, but it's not actually about us. It's not about fixing *ourselves*. Instead, God entrusts us in this way to partner with Him on behalf of someone else—either someone we know, or will come to know—who's dealing with the very thing we're experiencing. God may reveal answers to their physical problems through us or call us to intercede on their behalf.

It's easy to offer opinions and advice to people struggling with their health when we're on the outside looking in—when we don't fully *know* their struggles. It's an entirely different story to be immersed in their hardship through personal experience.

Years ago, when my nutrition practice was growing substantially, I noticed I was often physically experiencing what my patients were experiencing. At the time, I didn't think much about it beyond coincidence. But the more it happened, the more I paid attention.

The first time it happened, it was my gallbladder. Any consumption of fats and specific foods caused severe gallbladder and gastric pain along with a variety of other symptoms. The signs all pointed to gallbladder inflammation. I radically changed my diet and added in a specific supplement to address it and, as long as I was diligent, the pain subsided and my digestion gradually improved.

Much to my surprise, while still on my strict diet, a handful of new patients came to see me, all with gallbladder issues. *Well how convenient,* I thought. *I have firsthand experience to know what they're feeling and how to advise them more precisely.* In the whole endeavor, I felt like the Lord had pointed me to the very answers they needed.

Not long after that, my gallbladder normalized. I was able to return to a normal way of eating and discontinue the supplement.

The next time it happened, it was silent reflux. I didn't necessarily feel heartburn with the reflux, but developed a constant throat clearing tendency that was as annoying as a dripping faucet—both to me and my poor husband. Once I figured out that it was silent reflux, I adjusted my diet and supplements yet again and things calmed down. Wouldn't you know that suddenly I had a couple of new patients come in that had the exact same symptoms of silent reflux but didn't know what it was. Had I not experienced it myself, I would have completely missed it or perhaps assumed the cause to be something else with similar symptoms.

I advised my patients accordingly, knowing with near certainty this was the issue, and they both saw great reduction in their symptoms. Within a week or so, my nagging throat clearing went away, along with any other sign of silent reflux. I was able to eat the foods I had been avoiding, discontinue the supplement and, once again, all was well.

It's happened more times than I can remember over the years with patients, friends, and family members. I had no clue it was actually a supernatural thing until the first truly noteworthy experience got my attention. Out of nowhere, I began experiencing sporadic episodes of diarrhea. It hit me so suddenly and so severely that I had to bolt to the restroom. Not only was it extremely unpleasant and embarrassing, but I found myself hesitant to leave the house for fear of being stranded in public.

Eventually, I remembered to ask the Lord what this was and what was causing it. I thought about my diet and lifestyle—nothing had changed. I was eating as usual and was not stressed or anxious about anything. There were no other symptoms or issues—I was healthy in every way except for this.

A week into this unpleasant experience, I had a very strange dream. I saw Jesus as He was looking at another man, and He told the man, "It's the sugar." That was it.

When I woke up, I was deeply moved by the dream, sensing it was profound in some way. I asked the Lord to help me understand what it meant, but He didn't say much of anything and I didn't have any radical revelations. I decided to take the dream at face value and consider it in practical terms. Perhaps, "it's the sugar," meant sugar was the culprit behind these crazy bathroom issues I was having and, in the dream, Jesus was bluntly telling me so.

I tested my theory by removing all traces of sugar from my diet. With that, all diarrhea stopped. My body returned to normal with no further issue and, by God's grace, all was well again—except for the fact that I could no longer eat any amount of sugar.

The following weekend, a friend from college came to town for a short visit. It was 113 blistering degrees outside and any hope of being outdoors was gone. Thank God for air conditioning.

We putzed around the house for a while, and eventually decided to do some baking. I suggested we make a pie—yes, one with lots of yummy diarrhea-inducing sugar in it. Not my finest decision; I'm not really sure what I was thinking.

Despite our amateur skills, we made a peach pie that turned out beautifully. I prayed and asked God about eating it, hoping He would tell me to just eat and enjoy it with my friend, but He said nothing. Was this a moment where God would graciously protect my body and let me enjoy? Or was it a time when I needed to be disciplined and avoid it? When we sliced into the pie the next day, I decided to only have a sliver. Sure enough, within one minute of eating it, I bolted to the bathroom.

Ugh.

It seemed I now had a severe reaction to sugar and I was just going to have to stay away from it altogether. It wasn't the worst thing in the world to have to avoid, but something about it didn't sit well with me. You know my story. God had healed me and had always met any challenge to that healing with an answer.

I prayed for wisdom to know more about what this was. Suddenly my mind flashed back to the dream, and I remembered that Jesus wasn't talking to me. He was talking to another man and I simply observed it.

Finally, it clicked. *Oh! This isn't about me; it's for someone else.*

It took only a few minutes for me to know who that someone else was. I had an inkling that it was for a friend's husband. I called my friend and shared the dream with her, as well as what I thought it meant. She agreed that it was likely for her husband and committed to share it with him as soon as possible.

After that phone call, the diarrhea completely subsided for me. I tried eating sugar again and had zero problems with no problems since. It was done. Message delivered.

A few weeks later, we heard back from my friend about her husband. He had been having digestive issues and diarrhea much like what I had been experiencing, but even more severe. It had been going on for a while and, apparently, God had already spoken to him about eliminating sugar, but he hadn't yet listened. This man loves his sweets, and giving them up was no small feat. But hearing something like this straight from Jesus—twice—seemed to be all he needed. He agreed this message was from the Lord and proceeded to eliminate all sugar from his diet. That, in and of itself, was miraculous. As a result, his digestion improved immensely, his diarrhea issues subsided, and he felt much better overall—even lost a few pounds!

For months, he was diligent to avoid all sugar, and soon found that he quite enjoyed it. Once he did add sugar back in, his sweet tooth had greatly reduced and he needed far less to be satisfied when he ate it.

It's been nearly a decade of working with patients, and I couldn't count how many times I have experienced someone else's health issues. The most recent episode, probably the most intense, was what felt like a stomach ulcer. Oh, it was painful. I was flustered by the severe bloating, the intense pain after a cup of coffee, and the all-consuming nausea from any acidic foods. Alcoholic beverages were completely out of the question unless I wanted to be miserable and bedridden. Any trace of citrus or acid caused immense pain.

I was in a frenzy to figure it out and fix it, desperate to feel better. One thing after another had to be removed from my diet for me to function throughout the day. It took nearly two weeks of struggling before I even thought to ask Jesus for help. Why it sometimes takes me so long to remember to ask is beyond me.

About two weeks into my misery, I had a new patient schedule a consultation. I reviewed his forms and my jaw dropped. He had severe gastroesophageal reflux disease with a hiatal hernia, and every single symptom he listed matched what I was experiencing. As I read through his information, I sensed a strong and loving rebuke from the Lord:

"Why haven't you asked me for wisdom and understanding?"

So many emotions pulsed through me in that moment, the first of which was relief. I immediately knew that what I had been experiencing had been in anticipation of working with this man. And, awful as it sounds, I was thankful this wasn't "mine;" I wouldn't have to deal with this for years to come.

My relief then turned to conviction as I realized I hadn't been asking the Lord for wisdom like He had taught me to. I had resorted to fixing myself when it felt hard and when I felt so sick. Surely I had seen the faithfulness of the Lord in every step of my journey in the past; how could I forget so quickly?

I repented before Jesus, and my conviction then turned into a deep compassion for this patient. While I had been relieved that I wouldn't have to suffer with this forever, knowing God had allowed me to experience it for a time on behalf of someone else, my heart broke to realize this man had been dealing with it for twenty years.

Twenty years. I cried out to God for wisdom to offer this man—for answers, for healing, and for help.

When he and his wife came in for the initial consultation, I was even more amazed at just how exact his symptoms were to mine, from the grandest symptom to the smallest detail. I *literally* knew what he was feeling, what he was going through. He, too, had figured out how many things he had to avoid—things he loved—to function throughout the day and not be bedridden in pure misery. But even with these discoveries, he still suffered.

I asked the Lord what I was to do, and He simply asked me to pray for this man. Apart from that, I was just to advise him like I would any other patient, tending to his physical needs so his body could heal. I determined I would wait until the end of our appointment to pray so as to not jump the gun and make things too awkward too fast.

By the end of his first appointment, we had a good plan in place. We would run some additional tests, adjust several things in his diet, start him on some specific supplements, and go from there. He and his wife were Christians and had given me permission to counsel them through a Christian perspective so, as we were wrapping things up, I asked if I could pray for him. They were much obliged. It wasn't anything earth-shaking and profound, but I knew it was what God had asked me to do.

All of my symptoms left within the next few days. At his next visit, he reported a tremendous improvement with the changes and supplements. We reviewed his lab work, which helped me advise him on more specific changes to what he was eating and, three weeks later, he walked in a completely changed man. He was able to start drinking coffee again, as well as the occasional alcoholic beverage. Every symptom was completely gone and he felt amazing. He was elated; his wife was beyond thankful.

I couldn't thank the Lord enough. After just a glimpse of what this man had been through, I now knew the magnitude of his victory. Although he subsequently experienced a few setbacks, learning the balance between freedom and wisdom, he's still enjoying his improved health and continual progress.

Sharing in both His suffering and His victory taught me a great deal about the love of Jesus. When Jesus was nailed on that cross, He carried the pain and weight of both our sins *and our sicknesses*. Each time I experience someone else's health issues, bearing the weight of their pain, I try to remember that this is the very thing Jesus did for me. It's a great honor to learn the beauty of suffering love.

> "...'He took up our infirmities and carried our diseases.'"
> MATTHEW 8:17

> "As they led him away, they seized Simon from Cyrene, who was on his way in from the country, and put the cross on him and made him carry it behind Jesus."
> LUKE 23:26

Simon was a man forced to help Jesus carry his cross—his physical, wooden, immensely heavy cross. Jesus had already been betrayed, arrested, mocked, and severely flogged just short of death. He was suffering what no one could fathom, about to suffer even more, and now forced to carry a hundred pounds of wood on his back toward his death.

On His way to Golgotha, with soldiers on every side and loved ones following in tears, Simon passed by. Soldiers seized Simon. They pushed him behind Jesus and laid the cross upon him too. It took one verse to tell us about this moment, but can you fathom how long and agonizing that journey must have actually been? Simon followed behind Jesus the entire way. What did Simon think about as he felt the weight of the cross on his shoulders? Did he wince from the pain of the cross and the inconvenience of it? Or did the weight of the cross only make real the suffering that was being endured by Jesus in front of him?

No one had a greater glimpse into Jesus' suffering at that moment than Simon. If he was a praying man, I can only imagine what he might have been praying as he felt the weight with every step, saw the agony with every jolting turn, and knew he could only carry so much of this man's burdens. I wonder if Jesus felt the load lighten just slightly when Simon came to help. Maybe He felt a tiny fraction of relief in his last journey on earth to not be completely alone in His pain.

There is something ironically beautiful about the story of Simon and Jesus. Simon came behind Jesus and helped carry His cross, easing His burden just a bit, all while Jesus carried the weight of our burdens, sin, and shame when He was nailed to that cross.

When we are entrusted with experiencing someone else's health issues, it is a beautiful opportunity to fall in line behind them, to carry a little piece of their hardship or pain. When we feel their weight come upon us, may we find compassion well up inside us to its fullness.

Be discerning in how you steward such a priceless opportunity. What is the Lord asking of you to do with that cross? Sometimes He gives us answers for them, sometimes we are just there to help and pray and meet them with compassion along the way. It's not usually pleasant. It's not comfortable or easy. It is, however, an opportunity to intercede with greater authority, understanding, and insight. And, when the story is done, I pray you will stand in awe at the goodness of God and the honor of that with which you were just entrusted, much like Simon.

There is no love so deep, so profound, as a love willing to suffer for the sake of another.

chapter 22

a sound mind

> "When you discover something sweet, don't overindulge and eat more than you need, for excess in anything can make you sick of even a good thing."
>
> PROVERBS 25:16 (TPT)

Of all the reasons we might face health issues, one of the most obvious is poor eating habits. Perhaps it's eating too much food, or too much of certain foods and not enough of others. How we eat, what we eat, how much we eat, and when we eat are all governed by self-control. In a world where most of us have the luxury of having more than enough volume and variety of food, self-control is essential.

There are times when God wants to give us comfort through a cookie, celebration with a feast, or freedom to eat whatever is set before us but, in the midst of every one of those moments and all the days in between, self-control is paramount. We must recognize that our bodies still need to be cared for. They need good nutrition and proper fuel. The body doesn't thrive in a state of constant excess, lack, imbalance, or neglect. Wisdom and freedom also seek counterbalance: freedom needs the boundaries of wisdom.

Have you ever heard of the freshman fifteen? It refers to the fifteen pounds of weight gain that many freshmen in college experience. Why is this so common? Because, for many of these young adults, college life is their first step into full freedom in what they eat and how they live. They can eat whatever they want, whenever they want, and do whatever they want. Hopefully they'll adopt healthy habits, but it's up to them. There are no parents to cook for them, no chaperone to encourage them.

Freedom without self-control is dangerous. Self-control without freedom is stifling. So, how do the two coexist?

We can strive to obtain self-control through disciplines like dieting, portion control, food restrictions, and firm rules, but that's usually an ongoing battle that never seems to be won. Chronic dieting and unending restrictions pave the way for a mindset that always looks at food as the enemy.

Self-control is not something we accomplish as the result of extreme self-discipline, because self-control is a fruit of the Holy Spirit. This means that we can't obtain it and maintain it in our own strength; we need the Holy Spirit to help us.

> "For God gave us a spirit not of fear but of power and love and *self-control*."
> 2 TIMOTHY 1:7 (ESV, emphasis mine)

> "But the fruit of the Spirit is love, joy, peace, patience, kindness, goodness, faithfulness, gentleness, and *self-control*..."
> GALATIANS 5:22 (emphasis mine)

In the New King James Version, the term "self-control" is referred to as "a sound mind." This means that self-control is not just about discipline and rules. It's not about us controlling ourselves, but rather about seeing things rightly—seeing food rightly—with a sound mind.

Unhealthy mindsets permeate our health and nutrition culture. Even the healthiest people—by physical standards—have some of the most broken mindsets about food.

Remember that food is a gift meant for so many things beyond just health and sustenance. If we manage to do all the right things with our diet by certain nutrition standards, but still view food with an unhealthy mindset, then we are missing the sound mind that is the basis of godly self-control. A sound mind considers the heart and mind of God for food as well as the information and knowledge at hand. It doesn't over-exalt one thing at the expense of another. It filters all things through a lens of the Holy Spirit and what He is saying—using our powers of discernment to make decisions.

This battle for self-control is not merely a physical one—to eat, to not eat, or what to eat. It is one of both the mind and the spirit. Jesus says that the Holy Spirit gives us power and a sound mind, and that promise extends to our ability to eat with wisdom and healthy moderation in our day to day lives. We must lean into Him, seeking His help where our flesh feels powerless to avail.

Whether it is learning to eat better quality foods, eat more sensible portions, or something altogether different, we must ask for His help. We listen and then have a choice to make. We must choose to do our part in agreement by gradually making changes as there is grace to do so.

True self-control from the Spirit enables us to yearn for and crave what's good for us. It's not a constant denying of ourselves, our joy, or our freedom, but rather a divine transformation within us that stirs us to desire and crave what is good and life-giving for us. Quite simply, it's a change of heart as well as a change of mind.

God can give us the tools and strength we need to make good choices and the willpower to let go of foods or habits that are not wise. What if we could eat well because we wanted to? What if we actually enjoyed the foods that make us feel good? Isn't that a much better way?

One of my constant prayers is: *God, give me a sound mind. Help my body to crave the foods that it needs—the foods that are good and life-giving for me.* No more leaning on, "I should do this. I shouldn't do that."

We still have to intently choose the new and good cravings or ideas rather than staying with the easy and habitual but, with Him, there is help to do so. We have to choose to partner with God's help to make it effective.

One of my most challenging patients was completely transformed after we prayed for the Lord to help her in some of these more practical ways. She was, and still is, a very picky eater, set in her ways. Her living situation limited her ability to cook much and she didn't have any motivation or desire to figure out new strategies. As a result, she ate out for most meals and overindulged on a regular basis.

We hit wall after wall after wall with every dietary recommendation I made. Either she hated the foods I recommended or pushed back against new ideas because she didn't want to make the effort to try. I was, to be honest, growing quite frustrated and feeling at the end of my abilities. So, at her next consultation, I decided to pray with her before making one final round of suggestions. We prayed together for the Lord to help her body crave good things, and for just plain old *help* to be able to change. There was nothing profound about it—just a practical prayer enlisting the Lord's help.

A few days later, she had a powerful revelation from Jesus: specific things from her childhood had caused her to adopt unhealthy habits and become a very picky eater. With this revelation, she was finally able to understand why she was so stonewalled from change and why she felt compelled to consistently treat herself to really indulgent food. The understanding changed *everything*. She began craving different foods and found herself actually wanting to change. She decided it was finally time to put in the effort to try new things—things she had previously refused to try, recipes she'd refused to make. She tried them all and—wouldn't you know—she fell in love with most of them.

Gradually her entire way of eating transformed. She found herself not wanting any of the old foods she had clung to and became a huge fan of her new way of life. Her weight stabilized, and her severe gastrointestinal symptoms began to dissipate. We still had to pick and choose what things were realistic for her and what things were not, as her circumstances were still unique, but the ceiling that once held her back was gone. Everything radically changed after we enlisted the Lord's help.

Self-control may start with small victories but, eventually, it grows and bleeds into every part of our lives. When we gain a sound mind about food and health, we start to see the threads of that sound mind translate into other areas of life as well. It's no longer about right and wrong, do and don't. It's about the mercy and grace and goodness of God.

This, in turn, can radically change how we live—no longer being ruled by opinions, trends, and rules. We become less easily influenced, less easily swayed, less extreme in our opinions, because we strive to see it all through the mind of Christ. This is freedom. This is wisdom.

chapter 23

being human

I've seen God do some really amazing things with patients—hearts healed, people saved, demonic afflictions leaving, and miraculous healings—but, at the same time, many of my patients simply have broken bodies in need of physical answers.

We are human. Our bodies are incredible creations capable of more than we often realize. Every cell, pathway, organ system, bone, muscle, and tissue work together in beautiful unison to protect, heal, and sustain life. In this world, however, these bodies will malfunction, break, and wear out simply because it's a broken world and we aren't in heaven yet.

That's not to say that God won't supernaturally help us, but the cause, symptoms, and remedies may be straightforward. A cold might just be a cold. Digestive issues might stem from a broken system in need of repair. Nutrient deficiencies may be the byproduct of wear and tear on the body or a lack of nutrients in our diets. Our genes may be compromised. Disease may be the result of a vast array of compounding physical issues. Ultimately, we are human; not every health issue has a spiritual or emotional connection to search out.

How do you know when to look beyond the health issues for something deeper or when to take them at face value? My recommendation, as you step back and seek the Lord, is to always look at both. Don't ignore what's right in front of you, but be diligent to ask if there is anything deeper as well. It can be as simple as going through a quick check-in with the Holy Spirit. Ask the Lord questions. Do you sense something more going on in the spirit realm than you can see in the natural? Is there conviction for sin that you are ignoring? Are you going through a stressful time or dealing with difficult emotions? Overall, consider if there is anything that feels more significant about what you are experiencing than meets the eye. If, in the end, nothing gets highlighted and you don't feel the Holy Spirit tugging on you, then proceed with treating it as a purely physical issue until you know differently. The Lord may show you something down the road, so always be attentive, but don't overthink it. Don't get consumed with hunting for something that might not be there, just be faithful to ask and discern.

As Spirit-filled believers, we have to learn how to recognize what is happening in the spirit as much as we need the eyes on our face to see what's going on in the natural. We need to discern when God is speaking or highlighting something beyond the surface and when He isn't. Knowing when He isn't is just as important as knowing when He is.

Keep in mind that you might get it wrong. At some point, you probably will. I've gotten it wrong plenty of times. In those times, it's not really about being wrong, but being on a journey. Sometimes we can discern clearly right away; other times it's a process. Even if you take a wrong turn, Jesus is more than able to redirect you through it.

When the disciples asked Jesus about a man born blind, they searched for a spiritual reason for his blindness.

> "His disciples asked him, 'Rabbi, who sinned, this man or his parents, that he was born blind?' 'Neither this man nor his parents sinned,' said Jesus, 'but this happened so that the work of God might be displayed in his life.'"
>
> JOHN 9:2-3

It was well understood back then that infirmities could be the result of a person's sin. The disciples assumed as much with the blind man, but Jesus graciously informs them that they are wrong. This man's affliction had nothing to do with sin at all. He was simply blind. Yet there was a purpose to be found in the physical defect: that the glory of God would be displayed in his life.

What if, in every inexplicable health challenge, we could see an opportunity for the glory of God to be displayed? What if every sickness could be an opportunity to see Jesus to do something wonderful?

As we keep reading, we notice that Jesus didn't leave the man in his blindness.

> "…he spit on the ground, made some mud with the saliva, and put it on the man's eyes. 'Go,' he told him, 'wash in the Pool of Siloam.' So the man went and washed, and came home seeing."
>
> JOHN 9:6

The blindness was a physical infirmity, but Jesus healed him with supernatural provision and purpose.

Jesus spat on the ground and made mud to put on the man's eyes. But then He charged the man to wash in the Pool of Siloam. We see, once again, that Jesus does His part then prompts us to do ours—to take action in response to His voice.

When we are faced with health issues that are purely physical, it's still valuable to hear from the Lord. What is He saying? How is He leading? Or is He empowering us to take steps using our good judgment? If the disciples hadn't asked Jesus about the man's blindness, they would have never known what He would show them.

The Lord may lead us to practical answers–using natural remedies to help us heal. Or, He might answer with supernatural instructions that defy our logic or understanding—like He did with the blind man. Practical answers are no less powerful than supernatural ones—practical tools and natural remedies in the hands of the Almighty can be just as glorious and life changing. It's still His provision and His healing. After all, anything natural or tangible came from Him too.

I'm very certain that mud wasn't the typical remedy for blindness back then, nor is it now. It was, however, this man's remedy because of the blessing Jesus put on it. In the same way, we can ask that every step we take, every effort we make—be it practical or otherwise—would be supernaturally blessed and empowered to do more than it naturally should. If Jesus is breathing on it and blessing it, there is no limit to how effective it can be.

Your health journey is meant to carry the glory of God. That's a promise. What that means, is taking care of your body as you see fit and staying in step with Him as you do. Don't go where He isn't leading or where you don't sense His blessing. Also, remember to ask for His blessing. Pray over the steps you take and believe that the glory of God will come and be magnified through it all.

Keep in mind that the enemy may also try to lead you in a thousand wrong directions, trying to convince you it's the Lord. Remember, the Lord's ways are marked with peace, filled with hope, accompanied by good fruit, and are easily discerned by those who know Him. They are not heavy and burdensome but full of life.

Writing this book has been quite a journey—full of exhilarating moments of revelation as well as hard-fought battles. Time and time again, I've faced health issues that have caused me to put these truths to the test—growing evermore in my ability to discern and navigate what's happening with what the Lord is saying. I've experienced so many spiritual afflictions, so many prophetic afflictions, and so many symptoms stirred up by emotional stress that I can easily forget that sometimes my body just breaks because it breaks. It's easy to become like Jesus' disciples, always searching for some deeper understanding, unable to recognize the times when there is no deeper cause to search out.

A few years ago, I found myself constantly depressed, unmotivated, and unable to write. I also noticed some new skin issues that I had never dealt with before. The skin issues were annoying but not really a big deal. The depression and inability to write, however, were persistent and problematic. I was convinced that this was the enemy standing in my way once more. I prayed, declared truths, asked others to pray, and even fasted, but nothing helped. That supposed affliction never left.

A friend of mine, who is also an author, checked in to see how things were coming with the book. I told her about my struggles, attributing them to the enemy, and asked her for prayer. She emailed back, asking if nutrient deficiencies might be at play, or if changing my diet could help in some way.

I was *indignant*. Had she forgotten what I do for a living? I work with patients every day dealing with nutrient deficiencies and prescribing dietary changes for medical issues. Didn't she think I could recognize a nutrient or diet issue when I saw one? No. *This* was not *that*.

I was so lost in being offended at the gall of my friend to try to fix me rather than just pray for me that I never actually stepped back to consider whether she might be right.

Then, weeks later, I had a dream: a supplement bottle appeared before me with a specific nutrient name on the label. That was it. When I woke up, I instantly knew the Lord was showing me what my body was lacking, that this was a supplement I physically needed. What's funny is that, once I knew what nutrient I was missing, I knew exactly why I had been struggling and what was physically not working in my body. It made perfect sense.

I started on the supplement and, within a month, I was like a new person. I felt stable and grounded for the first time in a while, like a light switch had turned back on inside of me. I could think clearly and go about my daily tasks without feeling like I could barely put one foot in front of the other. Beyond that, several other symptoms that had been flaring up—the skin issues as well as some severe joint pain—all resolved with this nutrient as well. There was no way I could have connected all the dots without the Lord's intervention.

It turns out, my friend was right. I had spent so much time praying against the enemy, asking others to pray, believing it was a spiritual affliction, and all along it was purely something physical. The Lord never scolded me for getting it wrong, though I did have to repent for my pride and indignation towards my friend. He was so gracious and kind to answer me, even when I wasn't asking.

Since then, God has given me two other dreams about specific nutrients that I have needed for different reasons—one dream even included a specific dose to take. I never would have chosen these on my own, but they have made a world of difference in my physical health. His wisdom truly is better than mine.

Accepting that something is purely physical does not mean we are doomed to deal with it the rest of our lives. It doesn't mean that we will not see breakthrough or that the journey will be harder and longer. It just means that what we are facing is physical.

God isn't too big to help us find practical answers when we need them. Often, His answers are a lot simpler than we think. We just have to be humble enough to recognize His help when it comes.

This experience, and many others since, have taught me to stay flexible. Even when I think I know the source of my ailment or the crux of an issue, I must continually seek the Lord's help and pay attention. Humility and discernment are key. Sometimes it is simply a physical issue, but it's always an opportunity for God's glory to be revealed.

It may take time to get to the right answers for physical ailments, but Jesus doesn't rush through anything. He is thorough and intentional with us. There may be multiple layers to walk through, finding not just one right answer but many little ones that bring gradual healing along the way. You might find that your body heals quickly, or it may take time, perseverance, and patience. I'm convinced that delayed answers only serve to increase the degree of glory released when we finally get the breakthrough we need.

If you feel like there is something in your body that you need physical answers for, rest in knowing that the Lord wants you to find them more than you do. Seek His face. Follow His lead. Do the work. He is Jehovah Jireh, our faithful Healer.

chapter 24

from glory to glory

While healing is very much within God's ability and desire for us, our days are still numbered on this earth. A time will come when each of us will go home to be with Jesus, and sickness may simply be the vessel through which He brings us there.

> **"Precious in the sight of the Lord is the death of his saints."**
> PSALM 116:15

No one grieves our death from this world more than Jesus. Why, you might ask, would He grieve such loss more than you or me if our loved one dies? Especially if that loved one is going to heaven to be with Him? Jesus grieves because we grieve. He feels every ounce of heartbreak we feel in the wake of a precious saint's departure. He weeps because we weep. It doesn't matter that He knows the endgame and the glory that this person is now entering into. He willingly enters into our pain, feeling every last drop of it with us because He loves us.

Jesus knows every single person's grief. I wonder how painful that must be—my pain plus your pain, as well as everyone else's pain. And still, He chooses it and cherishes it. Compassion at its greatest.

After speaking at a women's retreat a few years ago, a lady came up to me struggling to understand her friend's recent health battle. Her close friend had suffered from severe heartburn and reflux. Eventually she ended up in the hospital as her health strangely declined from something that would not normally be life-threatening. Doctors could not give her much in the way of insight or answers; nothing seemed to make sense medically.

Her sick friend was fully convinced that God would heal her and, as her health declined, continuously reached out for healing prayer. She fought and fought for a miracle but, in the end, she passed away.

The lady asked me if I had ever heard of someone passing away from heartburn or reflux. I hadn't—and I have to wonder if there was more to the story as far as what was medically going on. Nonetheless, doctors never found answers. A good diet never provided healing. We will likely never know on this side of heaven what caused her death, but what bothered this woman most was why God didn't heal her friend.

This is a hard question to answer. Who of us knows the mind of God or can understand His ways? I hesitated to answer, not wanting to minimize the painful loss of her friend. Silently, I asked God for wisdom to know what to say. It wasn't a moment for platitudes or rationale; it was a moment where either God needed to speak or I needed to say nothing.

In the moment of silence, I heard the Holy Spirit whisper, "Sometimes there is a sickness that is intended unto death, and it is time for that person to come home." I paused for a moment to be sure this was right, then proceeded to share with her, hoping and praying it would be received well.

She was silent for a moment as she took it in. I could see her face and countenance start to soften as she thought about it this way. It appeared to reframe the entire understanding of her friend's defeat as one that was actually victorious in what it accomplished. Something so simple brought this woman great comfort. She thanked me with a gentle voice and walked away completely satisfied with the Lord's answer.

God's desire is always to heal—even when healing doesn't happen right away or hasn't happened yet. Even when the battle seems to have been lost in the defeat of death and the fullness of healing happens in heaven rather than on earth, He is our Healer. There is a time to contend for life, and there is a time to prepare our hearts for a passing to our glorious heavenly home.

The apostle Paul knew the difference between the two well. In the many years he spent serving the Lord, he faced death over and over, but it was not yet his time to go.

> **"...exposed to death again and again. Five times I received from the Jews forty lashes minus one. Three times I was beaten with rods, once I was stoned, three times I was shipwrecked, I spent a night and a day in the open sea, I have been constantly on the move. I have been in danger from rivers, in danger from bandits, in danger from my own countrymen, in danger from Gentiles, in danger in the city, in danger in the country, in danger at sea; and in danger from false brothers."**
>
> 2 CORINTHIANS 11:23-26

Every time I read these verses, I think: *Okay, I'll never complain again.* No matter what he faced, he persevered because there was still purpose for his life on earth. He knew God was bigger than those obstacles, even though they were pretty big ones.

Then the time came. Paul had fulfilled all that the Lord had put in his heart to do. It was nearing his time to die, and he knew it. Because of that, he was able to walk through it with tremendous peace and anticipation.

> **"For I am already being poured out like a drink offering, and the time has come for my departure. I have fought the good fight, I have finished the race, I have kept the faith. Now there is in store for me the crown of righteousness, which the Lord, the righteous Judge, will award to me on that day—and not only to me, but also to all who have longed for his appearing."**
>
> 2 TIMOTHY 4:6-8

Paul knew when a trial was something he had to persevere through and when his time on earth was complete. Because of this, he did not lay down and give up prematurely. He did not assume anything by circumstances alone, but he knew these things by the Holy Spirit and revelation from the Lord. Death was not the end for him. It was his highest goal since the moment he radically encountered Jesus on the road to Damascus. He lived his life in pursuit of the one to come and, because of this, death did not threaten him.

Each of us will depart from this temporary world at one time or another. Sometimes it comes suddenly and, at other times, like Paul, we are given the opportunity to know it's coming. Any person facing a sickness that may lead to death needs the freedom to process this with the Lord themselves. They may respond like Hezekiah—grieved and compelled to cry out to the Lord for mercy, that He may change His mind and add more years to their life. Or, like Paul, they may wrestle only to find peace in knowing they have fulfilled all that they needed to accomplish in this life, and it's time for them to go home.

It's not usually simple or easy—death never is. Paul didn't have a wife, children, or other complexities of saying goodbye that many of us would face. His life on earth was impossibly hard, and it's only fitting that he longed for his heavenly home. Either way, whether it is easy to accept or agonizing and painful, Jesus is there in the midst of our grief, carrying it with us. Precious in His eyes are the deaths of His beloved saints.

> **"...the righteous are taken away to be spared from evil. Those who walk uprightly enter into peace; they find rest as they lie in death."**
>
> ISAIAH 57:1-2

Our journey isn't supposed to culminate in one singular moment of perfect health. Moments of victory are important and powerful; Solomon speaks of those moments saying, "a longing fulfilled is a tree of life." But our ultimate longing is for Him and for our home. Our happily ever after lies in heaven.

PART FOUR

the river of life

chapter 25

two rivers

From the moment I cried out to God nearly ten years ago asking Him for a better way, He has shown me more than I could have imagined. What stands out most is that everything hinges on the greatness of His love. Every story, every lesson, every revelation I have shared with you is a testimony of His love.

Food is delicious, moments around food are special, and healing is awesome but, tie all those to the God of all creation, and it's His love through them that will minister to the depths of our souls. It's His love that will give us joy, comfort, connection, or healing. It's His love that will enable us to persevere, to hope, to believe for more than we can presently see.

He is faithful to transform our journeys and our experiences with food into something profoundly special and victorious. My hope and prayer for each of you reading this book is that you will see everything in a new way. Whether it's food, moments around food, or health, I pray you would see it all through the lens of how deeply the Father and our Savior love you and long to bless you.

Three years into writing this book, the Lord gave me a vivid dream. From high up above, I saw a vast, muddy, dark river with a ferocious current. In the midst of the heavy current were scores of people being helplessly swept away.

Along the sides of the river, the current was less intense. It was there that I noticed a man clinging onto the edge to avoid being swept away. I watched as he pushed off the side of the riverbank and out into the raging waters, grabbed a person, and helped him or her navigate out of the current and over to the side. Once there, they grabbed on in relief as he then launched back out to help others. He did this over and over again, eagerly trying to save people from the current. Yet, in all his efforts, he never got anyone out of the muddy river, just out of the ferocity of the rushing waters.

With each person that was now latched onto the side of the river, there was relief. They no longer felt like they were going to drown, but soon they realized that there was also no further hope of escape. Despite feeling rescued, there they remained—in the dark, muddy waters—not knowing how to get out, or even that life beyond this river was possible. What initially felt like a rescue only went so far until they realized they were still waiting for something more, without knowing what, if anything, was possible. They longed for fullness of life while merely surviving.

At first glance, this man seemed to be helping these people. He believed he was; yet I heard the Lord's voice above me boldly declare, "He doesn't need to be in the water to help them."

I was confused. Wasn't he helping them out of the heavy current? Wasn't that a good thing?

I woke up from the dream amazed by what I had witnessed; but what did it all mean? Rivers usually represent the Spirit or presence of God throughout the scriptures, the place where life is found and healing comes. Yet I had a keen sense that this river was not of God and it was not good. The muddy dark appearance alone suggested something was wrong. It was sweeping people away to destroy their lives, not to give life.

I thought about it for a while, knowing it was profound and important, but couldn't make sense of it. A few days later, as I wrote the dream out in my journal, the Lord's voice came so abruptly, mid-sentence, and with such incredible urgency, that I nearly gasped out loud.

"It's the *wrong river*. My people are in *the wrong river*—the wrong current."

I could feel the Lord's presence surrounding me as His words sank in. Every piece started to make sense.

Our health and nutrition culture has become like this muddy river. It's overwhelming us, robbing us of life, of hope, of joy, and of the ability to see clearly. Our hearts are dying for lack of life.

The man in the river represented all the physical answers out there to help us—whether it's diet, supplements, lifestyle, or other therapies. These can, in fact, help us out of the heavy current but, by themselves, they have no power to get us out of that muddy river. They can only take us so far.

When we don't partner with the Lord in our health, when we don't view food through a lens of His love, there is no hope. Where there is no hope, there is no life. Darkness, confusion, heaviness, and frustration will try to overtake us because the enemy knows that robbing us of life in one area cripples other parts of our lives as well.

This book, this message, is not just about food or physical health. It's about our destiny as children of God. We have to believe God is who He says He is and that He will do what He says He will do in *all* areas of our lives. So many Christians know the Father, the Son, and the Holy Spirit deeply, but this part of their lives is like an appendage cut off from the life flow of the heart. If a part of us—any part of us—is disconnected from the heart of the Father, then we will never fully step into who we are called to be. It's as though we are living with an arm that doesn't function in unison with the rest of the body. That arm isn't simply not helping, it's hindering what the rest of the body is doing.

If we surrender to a lifeless journey—trudging forward in our own strength and left to our own devices—it will impact every part of who we are. Instead of being full of joy, hope, faith, and peace, it will pull the life right out of us. Not physical life or death, but spiritual.

It's time for our hearts to be resurrected.

Once I understood the muddy river, I began poring through scripture to remember what the river of God was like. It was different from the muddy river in every way.

> **"Then the angel showed me the river of the water of life, flowing with water clear as crystal, continuously pouring out from the throne of God and of the Lamb. The river was flowing in the middle of the street of the city, and on either side of the river was the Tree of Life, with its twelve kinds of ripe fruit according to each month of the year. The leaves of the Tree of Life are for the healing of the nations."**
> REVELATION 22:1-2 (TPT)

Consider the trees thriving on either side of the river of life, the ones that produce healing to the nations. The prophet Jeremiah said that these very trees represent those of us who trust in the Lord.

> **"But blessed is the man who trusts in the Lord, whose confidence is in him. He will be like a tree planted by the water that sends out its roots by the stream. It does not fear when heat comes; its leaves are always green. It has no worries in a year of drought and never fails to bear fruit."**
> JEREMIAH 17:7-8

Our confidence isn't meant to be in ourselves or in food, but rather in the faithfulness of God. As we look to Him and trust Him, we drink from the river of life.

When I started on my health journey, I found physical answers that helped. I grew in knowledge and understanding to fix my body and I became successful at helping others do the same. For a long time, I felt confident in these things—in nutrition, in functional medicine, in equipping people with knowledge and tools to fix their bodies.

This was good, but it wasn't complete; I was still missing something. That's when I had to shift my confidence from the tools I had over to the God of all creation who created both me and the tools. Over time, I got to know His character and realized that I could be confident in Him, in His voice, and in His faithfulness. I could partner with Him, rather than leaning on my own strength and understanding alone, to see far greater things unfold.

> **"Trust in the Lord with all your heart and lean not on your own understanding; in all your ways acknowledge him, and he will make your paths straight. Do not be wise in your own eyes; fear the Lord and shun evil. *This will bring health to your body and nourishment to your bones."***
>
> PROVERBS 3:5-7 (emphasis mine)

It's normal to search for tangible answers. In fact, it's not wrong. But that's simply not all there is available for us. The only thing that pulls us out of the muddy waters of this world is learning to trust the Lord and partner with Him.

Jesus often refers to us as sheep and Himself as our Shepherd. Herds of sheep can become so intimately accustomed to their shepherd's voice that they will not follow any other voice. That voice is the only one they trust to lead them to food, to protect them from harm, and to help them navigate terrain. It's how they were created—to depend on their shepherd. We, too, have the opportunity to get to know our Shepherd's voice and to trust Him to lead us in paths of life.

Life is contagious. When our spirits are full of life, it oozes out of us and impacts those around us. As such, our journey with food will impact those around us just as powerfully as it will transform us within. This is part of our destiny—to bear fruit continually and, in doing so, to change the world.

It's time for us to believe God for a better way—the way of His Kingdom—where anything is possible; where hope, health, and freedom abound.

chapter 26

redeeming food

Food was always meant to be a gift and a blessing from our Creator, a plumb line that connects us to the very heart of the Father. It was meant to give us life and cultivate life-giving things in and around us. As with any good thing, we can miss it. We can over analyze it, mishandle it, misunderstand it, abuse it, pervert it, or despise it. It can be turned from something intended to bless into something that feels more like a curse—robbing us of life rather than filling us. But that doesn't mean it can't be redeemed and restored back to the very gift it was created to be.

Jesus wants to redeem the gift of food for us, His bride. He wants to redeem our hearts to see it rightly so that it can be the blessing it was created to be. He wants us to love food the way He loves food, to experience the fullness of its beauty in every facet of our lives—the beauty that ultimately reflects Him and His love for us.

In the end, when our lives are over, we will remember moments with food that were dear to us, but not because of the food itself. We'll remember because of everything that happened around it— who we were with, the circumstances, the season, what our hearts experienced.

Food is merely a vessel for greater things.

As with any gift, we have to learn wisdom to know how to steward it well. As the Lord redeems our minds toward food, we need to fight to keep it redeemed. It's easy to go back to the muddy river—leaning on our own strength, our own understanding, our own devices—but instead let's intentionally choose to look to Jesus and His wisdom, staying always in the river of life.

We have a good Father who gives His children good things. Food is His gift to us, and it is good.

appendix

SALVATION: WHO IS THIS JESUS?

If you have never put your faith in Jesus, there is no better time than today. Who is He, you might ask? Jesus is the Son of God and the Savior of the world. When sin entered into the world, it disconnected us from the presence of our holy God. The wage of our sin is death, but Jesus was God's plan for redemption.

Jesus came to the world born of a virgin, and he lived as a mortal man. He lived a perfect life, without blemish, despite the many trials He endured. While He lived in this world, He performed many miracles and taught people about the kingdom of God that exists beyond what we physically see.

When the time came, Jesus gave His life for us. He suffered unimaginable pain at the hands of some of the very people He came to save. They nailed Him to a cross and mocked Him until, at last, He died. In death, He went to hell and endured unimaginable pain and darkness but, three days later, He rose. He came back to life from the grave, conquering death once and for all. Why did He give His life? It was payment for ours—our atonement. His sacrifice paid for our sins so that we could be forgiven and made holy once more. This is how God created us to be before sin entered into the world. His resurrection from the grave then accomplished for us eternal life.

When we acknowledge Jesus for all He did and put our faith in Him, our hearts become pure and we are promised an eternal life in the glory of His presence. Imagine everything good in this world in its perfect and purest form, where evil no longer exists, nor disease, nor death. This is eternity with the Lord.

Being forgiven and redeemed doesn't mean we live perfectly. It simply means that, whenever we mess up, forgiveness awaits us time and time again.

More than that, when we put our faith in Jesus, we get the privilege of then being filled with His Holy Spirit—the Spirit of God living inside us. We can commune with Him, learn to hear what He is speaking, and know what is on His heart. We can live full of light, with His joy as our strength, and we can walk in His power. The darkness of this world no longer has a grip on us when we put our faith in Jesus because greater is the Savior who lives in us than the enemy who rules over this broken world.

If you've never given your life to Jesus, I invite you to do so now. Ask Him to forgive your sins. Tell Him that you believe He is who He says He is, that He is your Savior who died so you might live. Invite His Spirit to come live inside you, to baptize you with His love and His power. Then, let His presence wash over you and make you new. Let Him refresh you inside and out, and embrace the new life He puts inside you.

Next, connect with other Christians. We aren't meant to navigate this world on our own; we need one another. Together we all make up the church—the Body of Christ.

As you get to know Jesus, be sure to find a Bible. The Word of God is our lifeline to knowing Father God and Jesus more intimately. His Words are full of life and hope.

Above all, get excited, because the journey with Jesus is worth more than you could ever imagine.

God bless you!
Laura Woodard, R.D., C.L.T.